THE CANDIDA DIET BOOK

KAREN BRODY is a freelance writer who writes mostly on health issues. In 1990 she was diagnosed as having candida and consequently changed her diet dramatically.

She has been a student at the Natural Gourmet Cookery School in New York, where she studied the relationship between food and healing and how to cook for special diets.

She has lived all over the world and currently resides in the United States with her husband.

Overcoming Common Problems Series

For a full list of titles please contact
Sheldon Press, Marylebone Road, London NW1 4DU

Overcoming Common Problems Series

Overcoming Common Problems Series

Overcoming Common Problems

THE CANDIDA
DIET BOOK

Karen Brody

sheldon PRESS

First published in Great Britain in 1997 by
Sheldon Press, SPCK, Marylebone Road, London NW1 4DU

Second impression 1998

British Library Cataloguing in Publication Data
A catalogue record for this book is available from the British Library.

ISBN 0–85969–761–4

Photoset by Deltatype Limited, Birkenhead, Merseyside
Printed and bound in Great Britain by
Biddles Ltd, Guildford and King's Lynn

Contents

Acknowledgments

Thanks to so many people involved with candida who openly spoke with me about this subject, sent me useful material and welcomed the idea of a new diet book on candida. I was overwhelmingly impressed by everyone's selfless desire to find ways for candida sufferers to feel better.

I thank Heidi Fleiss, chiropractor, kinesiologist and now friend, who provided the key to opening my door to a new, healthier diet.

I thank my surrogate brother and friend, Tyrone Sullivan, for his information and demonstration of how successful a 'theme' meal can really be.

I thank my 84-year-old grandmother, Madaline – a dietician by training – who loves wholefoods and chatting for hours with me about food and healing.

And thanks to my Mom, who still hates tofu, and whose speciality for dinner is to order a Chinese take-away, but none the less, has tried countless candida meals and said she cannot believe how good they taste. Your love, support and trips to Mana restaurant have always been appreciated.

I thank Tim, for his continued love through the years; for getting excited about a diet that initially seemed crazy; for changing the brown rice to millet when I decided at the last minute that my body did not want brown rice; and for believing in me, always.

Finally, I thank my Dad, a very mainstream man, who I only now realize had a lot of courage when he decided to heal himself through food and meditation. Watching him, and his supportive partner, Jeanne, go on a very strict healing diet together was the strongest act of love I can imagine.

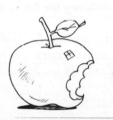

For Tim, with love

Introduction

'When illness arises, stop, look, and listen!'
   Dr Elson M. Haas, *Staying Healthy With the Seasons*

Food as fuel

Imagine your body is a car. When a car is full of the right fuel, it runs smoothly. If you put 2 star petrol into a car that only runs on 4 star, the car will become sluggish and perform poorly. The same is true about your body. If you put the right food in, you run smoothly. The wrong food could cause havoc.

A person with candida fits perfectly into this analogy. When you eat certain foods that the candida likes to feed on – like bread, sugar, and mushrooms – your body will feel sluggish and a multitude of unpleasant symptoms could occur. These foods are the wrong fuel for your body. By eating a diet of foods that do not feed the candida – one that includes fresh vegetables and grains – the candida has nothing to feed on and so you soon gain the potential to feel better. These foods are the right fuel for your body.

As you read through this book, you will discover that food is a very powerful tool for healing yourself. We eat food every day, yet rarely do we *stop, look and listen* to what food is doing to our body. Ignoring the crucial role of food in maintaining good health could have led to your current physical dis-ease. I intentionally hyphenate the word 'disease' in various places throughout this book to remind you that contracting a dis-ease is your body's way of saying it is no longer at ease. With the right food in your body, often combined with other therapeutic approaches, your body can regain the strength to feel 'at ease' again.

My story

Five years ago – after going to countless doctors for migraines, panic attacks, tingling in my shoulder, hands and feet – I ended up at the office of my friend's cousin, Heidi, a chiropractor and kinesiologist. I almost cancelled my appointment that day, sceptical that anything not involving a medical prescription would work, and too afraid of just physically getting to her office.

At the last moment, I jumped into a taxi and went. I felt so low and had lost hope, assuming after going to doctor after doctor that my multisymptomatic problems meant I either had a terminal illness or I had gone crazy. My initial visit with Heidi lasted two hours. I almost threw up on her twice. Naturally, I assumed the worst.

'You have something called candida,' she said with confidence. 'It's an overgrowth of yeast in your body.'

'Why has this happened?', I asked.

'There are many reasons. The fact that you have been on antibiotics continually for a year and a half is definitely one good reason.'

'So what do I do?' I said, expecting to be given another prescription.

'Go home and have a carrot juice, eat millet and wear orange. And stop all medication. We'll talk about your new dietary requirements tomorrow.'

I left her office thinking she was a freak. Have a carrot juice, eat millet and wear orange? What kind of a treatment was that? How could food make me feel better? I had been in a healthfood shop before, but it always felt like I was a visitor rather than going in there with the intention of buying something. Confused about her diagnosis and method of treatment, but feeling so deathly awful I would try anything, that night I bought millet and carrot juice at a healthfood shop and dug out the only piece of orange clothing I owned. To my surprise, my body felt calmer than it had in months.

The next day, Heidi gave me a list of foods I should and should not eat to help the candida clear up. I was in shock – everything I was currently eating I could no longer eat. My life felt like it had been flipped upside down. 'I'm sorry,' I barked at Heidi, 'but I don't cook, I don't have any time to cook, and I definitely do not know how to cook these strange foods.'

With a smile on her face she said, 'Go buy yourself a cookbook.

Any cookbook that feels right for you.'

I did and it changed my life.

I must admit, though, that I never would have found the motivation to change my diet if I had not felt so ill. To feel bad every day and have all the doctors tell you they do not know why feels like a punishment. At night I even cried out, 'I want to die! Please let me die!' So, when Heidi told me to change my diet and I would feel better, out of desperation I thought, what do I have to lose? Nothing, really.

While talking to many candida sufferers for this book, I discovered my experience was not uncommon. Many people recounted horror stories to me about endless visits to their unsympathetic doctor, bathroom cabinets full of prescription drugs, panic attacks while driving, eating out or shopping, not wanting to get out of bed in the morning, feeling like death was just around the corner. Their road to good health sometimes came only after much trial and error in trying to find the right approach for them.

Changing to a new healthier diet

This book will tell you what to eat when you have candida, but this is only one step in your new dietary regimen. You also have to know how to cope on a candida diet. How do you introduce new foods into your diet like soya milk and rice cakes, and give up foods like biscuits and coffee? Where is yeast hiding in some of the most common foods we eat? How can you get your family and friends to try the same foods you eat?

There are many strict dos and don'ts on this diet to starve the candida that is thriving in your system, but following these rules does not have to make it the worst experience of your life. As nutritionist Penny Davenport told me, 'The good news is a candida diet is actually very, very healthy. And, if people stick to it, they will feel better.'

It's true, you will feel better on this diet. Once the yeast begins to die – for some that will be a few months, for others it will be longer – your life will change. Countless numbers of former candida sufferers have said, 'It is like a cloud lifting in your head.'

Candida specialists stress that if you do not change your diet, you will not get rid of the candida. You can take antifungals, probiotics, vitamins and try many other natural remedies, but none of these alone will get you better – you also must change your diet.

Is a candida diet different for women, men or children?

The key to being on a successful candida diet – no matter what your age or sex – is to design your own personal daily eating regimen, bearing in mind the candida diet guidelines provided in this book and your personal needs. For example, most men need more to eat for lunch than a salad. Some experts also suggest that men eat more animal protein foods, while women should eat more vegetables. Diet expert Annemarie Colbin says this is perhaps because men discharge protein, carbohydrates and minerals faster than women, who tend to build up matter in their bodies.

Everyone has a different body, with different needs. The food one person can eat may not be what another person can tolerate. Likewise, the amount of food one person eats may not be the right amount for another. Honour your unique eating needs, using the guidelines provided in this book. Good health *is* just around the corner.

1
What is candida?

'If the immune system is healthy the growth of the candida can be kept under control; if it is not healthy, having been weakened by some prescribed drugs, such as antibiotics or steroids, or if resistance is low through poor nutrition, excessive alcohol, stress, illness or pollution, then the yeast can grow to such an extent that it interferes with normal body chemistry and can cause widespread baffling symptoms.'

Shirley Trickett, *Coping with Candida*

As you are reading this book, you have probably been told you have a condition called candida. Finally, a reason for all your aches and pains, PMS, fatigue, irritable bowel and other conditions. Initially, you feel relief – 'I knew it wasn't all in my head'. You go home to tell your family the diagnosis. 'Candida?', they say. They have never heard of it. You try to explain it, but they still don't get it.

When I was writing this book, I spoke to a woman with candida who told me she was also a coeliac. 'I was so happy to be a coeliac,' she said 'because everyone knows and accepts that diagnosis. People didn't laugh because they understood what it was. You can refuse foods and say it is because you are a coeliac.' It is true, explaining to your family and friends that you have candida can be quite difficult because people have not heard of it.

While candida is not as commonly understood by the general public as coeliac disease at present, thankfully more and more people are at least becoming aware that candida exists. Books are cropping up everywhere, and even a few enlightened GPs are recognizing candida and referring their patients to nutritionists. Candida is a multisymptomatic condition, fully explained in the companion to this book, *Coping with Candida* by Shirley Trickett. What follows is a brief overview of candida.

How candida grows in your gut

Candida albicans is a common yeast that lives in the body. Many yeasts live in the body, not just candida. When the immune system is strong, the candida is harmless. But when it is weak, from overuse of antibiotics, the Pill and various other environmental phenomena, the candida begins to multiply. For most people, when the immune system is weak, you go to your doctor and take antibiotics, thinking this will strengthen your immunity. If you use antibiotics for a long time, though, this will encourage the candida to grow and weaken your immune system. This overgrowth of candida emits toxins that weaken your immune system further. As a result, you get chronically sick and usually end up taking more antibiotics, which starts the cycle again.

By this time, the candida is thriving in your body, it is changing shape and growing whiskers, which resemble mould on bread. In this form, it can move through the wall of the intestine and into the bloodstream, placing itself anywhere in the body. This is known as a 'leaky gut'. Candida can get into the muscles, joints – virtually anywhere. When it does, most candida sufferers say they feel 'ill all over'. Then, allergies to food, chemicals, almost anything, are common as the immune system is now so weak it cannot fight back.

How do you know if you have candida?

Never self-diagnose. Many practitioners exist who can help you confirm whether or not candida exists and decide what treatment is right for you (see the Useful addresses at the back of this book). There are, however, two things you can do on your own to determine if candida might be causing your ill health.

Examine your personal history

Ask yourself the following questions.

- Have I ever been on antibiotics for a long period of time? This includes wide-spectrum antibiotics and drugs for acne.
- Have I been on the Pill or had HRT (hormone replacement therapy) for over six months?

- Have I been on medication for asthma, eczema or rheumatoid arthritis for a long period of time?
- Have I been on NSAIDs (non-steroidal anti-inflammatory drugs – usually given for back pain, arthritis, migraine, gout and menstrual problems)?
- Is my diet high in sugar, preserved foods, dairy products, foods that contain yeast (breads, Marmite), stimulants and depressants (coffee and diet coke) and low in fresh vegetables and whole foods?
- Do I sleep well at night?
- Am I experiencing any stress in my life?

If you answered 'yes' to several of these questions, especially the first five, then you may have candida.

Write down your symptoms

Everyone's body is different to the next person's and each manifests disease in its own unique way. As you now know, when candida takes hold, it can spread anywhere. For some it will go into the joints, for others it will travel into the bowel and for others it will go somewhere else, but it often spreads to several different areas.

The symptoms that identify candida also vary from person to person. In the list below are some of the most common symptoms candida sufferers experience. Yours may be different, but often you will have one or more of the following:

- persistent vaginal and oral thrush
- menstrual cramps, severe PMT, infertility
- irritable bowel syndrome
- skin conditions – acne, eczema, rashes, itching, athlete's foot
- food allergies or intolerances
- cold hands and feet, chilliness
- panic attacks
- depression, mood swings
- a fuzzy head
- ear, nose, throat and chest problems.

Why me and not my relative or friend who eats a less healthy diet than me?

When I was first diagnosed with candida, I could not understand why I – who did not eat a perfect diet but usually ate non-sugared cereals and a few fresh vegetables now and again – had candida and my brother – who lived on sugar-filled processed foods and did not seem to know what a fresh vegetable looked like – felt great and did not have candida. This made no sense and certainly didn't seem fair.

Now the answer is quite clear. Good health depends on your immune system. Some people have stronger immune systems than others. There are many reasons for this. Environment, whether you were breastfed as a child, how much junk food you had as a child – these are just some of the factors that shape the immune system.

It is also important to consider personality. Some people, regardless of whether they possess a cheerful or sad disposition, have the ability to let things go. Others do not.

The idea that the mind can influence the body has been gaining more and more attention because studies show that this relationship is true in so many circumstances. When we ignore our minds, we ignore our bodies. Everyone has a different relationship between their mind and body, thus a different immune system and different reactions to food. Acknowledge that it feels unfair if your health suffers from food allergies when so many other people around you do not. Then let that feeling go, knowing that you are who you are and they are who they are.

Taking action to feel better

Now that you know the causes and symptoms of candida and you are fairly certain you have it, you must make up your mind: do you want to feel better? This may seem like a silly question, because of course, intellectually, you want to feel better, but what is at the root of the question is another – are you ready to be actively involved in making yourself better? Doing this is the only way you will get rid of the candida. A pill won't do it; neither will an injection.

Three active steps you should take if you have Candida

First, see your doctor to get a complete physical examination. If they find nothing wrong, tell them you think you might have candida. If they do not believe you, thank them for their time, do not accept a prescription for your pain, and leave.

Second, go to see a reputable natural health practitioner. There are many practitioners – nutritionists, clinical ecologists, kinesiologists – skilled in treating candida patients (see also the Useful addresses section at the back of this book). They will most likely put you on antifungals and probiotics and suggests other supplements that suit your body. They will also insist you begin a candida diet.

Third, start on your candida diet. This is the one treatment for candida you cannot afford to pass on. All the experts agree, you will not get better if you do not change your diet. No one *wants* to change their diet, it even seems impossible at first, but once you get started and plan what you will eat and know what to buy, it does get easier. And it can actually be fun!

So, let's get started.

2

What foods you need to heal

'Let thy food be thy medicine and thy medicine be thy food.'
Hippocrates, over 2,500 years ago

The limits of modern medicine

Your health is in your own hands. Modern medicine can be useful
to some extent, but it has limits. Consider this scenario. Jane goes
to her doctor because she has been getting headaches. Her doctor
prescribes a drug that gets rid of the headache, but causes nausea.
She then takes another drug to counterattack the nausea, but that
irritates her stomach. For one year, she lives on antacid pills to
relieve her stomach ache. Eventually she goes back to her doctor
who refers her to a consultant who finds that she has developed an
ulcer, for which she takes medication. She continues to eat the
same diet she has always been on, foods loaded with sugar and lots
of dairy products. The medication relieves some of her discom-
fort, but she still finds she has to rely on antacids. One year later,
still complaining of a 'funny tummy' to her doctor, it is suggested
she might be suffering from anxiety and might want a drug to
relieve the anxiety.

Jane's health is out of control. Neither she nor her doctor is in
control of it any more. She is not getting better and, at best, will
just continue to feel bad unless she grabs the reigns. Many people
who have candida will be very familiar with Jane's scenario.
Remember, though, you *can* take control of your health.

Annemarie Colbin, author of the book *Food and Healing*, says
she sees three major errors in the assumptions we make about
health and illness today. They are:

- the belief that our physical symptoms (headaches, pimples,
  fevers) are erroneous reactions of the body to normal stimuli

10

- the belief that having surgery or taking a chemical substance, whether of natural or artificial origin, can restore health by interrupting the process called 'disease'
- the belief that dietary habits are unrelated to symptoms or illnesses.

All three of these are important to consider when you are trying to restore your health. You must get to know your body, listen to the subtle indications it gives you that add up to that 'I don't feel well' feeling and learn what unique methods your body needs to heal. A doctor cannot do the work for you to become healthy.

The importance of food in healing

The body hates imbalance. When you cut yourself, the body quickly restores its balance by forming a scab, which eventually falls off and the skin returns to normal. In a similar way, eating good food will create a feeling of balance, allowing the immune system to spend its time healing. Too much bad food will send the body off-balance, halting its natural instinct to heal. When we lack balance in our lives – whether it is physical, emotional or mental – we often feel bad physically. A good diet is one crucial step towards feeling better.

Many people have studied the effects of food and its ability to make us feel good and bad. In Kristina Turner's *Self-healing Cookbook*, she makes it very clear that food and mood are directly related. She says certain foods nurture different organs, and thus can produce different effects in the body. For example, eating grains like rye, barley, wheat and quinoa all help cleanse the liver and gallbladder, producing a patient, flexible feeling in your mood. Some foods are more likely to cause disease, like dairy products, which have been linked to so many female gynaecological problems. In moderation, any food may be OK, but studies show that our contemporary society does not eat in moderation any more. If you combine our poor diets with the amount of chemicals going into the air, food and water, it is not too surprising

11

that immunological diseases like cancer and asthma are rampant today.

If you have candida, your body is out of balance. The key then, like any dis-ease, is to bring it back into balance. Thinking about what you eat, how it will make you feel and what it will do to your body, will help restore your body into the healthy state it wants to be in.

Foods candida sufferers should and should not eat

The biggest complaint I have heard from people with candida is that each book on candida suggests something different to eat. One says 'yes' to eat some sugars, like fruit, and others say absolutely 'no' to fruit. Obviously, this is very confusing. My best advice is to choose a candida diet from one book, or your health practitioner's advice and diet sheet, and stick with it. Do not overwhelm yourself with the contradictions you see in all the different books. These contradictions exist mainly because, like any disease, what is right for you will be individual to you. Everyone has different bodies and different degrees of candida. If your friend, who also has candida, can eat one piece of fruit every week, but you can't, just remember that we are all different. You need to design a diet that is right for you, which is precisely the point of this book.

Foods to avoid

Candida likes to feed on sweet and fermented or yeast-containing foods – often the foods you are craving if you have candida. When you begin a candida diet, most experts insist you avoid a large number of the foods that feed the candida for at least three to four months. Depending on your condition, after this time period you could ease up a bit. Remember, especially in the beginning, if you follow the diet only 75 per cent of the time, you will still be feeding the candida. It will not die. Natural supplements used to kill the yeast will help, but they cannot do *all* the work in your body – you must clean up your immune system by not eating foods that make you feel bad. Diet expert Annemarie Colbin points out, 'Often it is not just what we eat, but also what we don't eat, that helps us become healthy again'.

The major foods you must avoid are:

- *all foods containing yeast* – Marmite, bread, pizza
- *all foods containing sugar* – most common breakfast cereals, puddings, honey, syrups, chocolate, biscuits, all canned drinks, most tinned vegetables and products with malt
- *all foods containing cow's milk* – cow's milk, cheese and cream
- *all fermented foods and drinks* – alcohol, foods containing vinegar (ketchup, pickles, baked beans), soy sauces
- *all foods containing fungi and mould* – mushrooms, nuts that are not fresh (nuts still in their shell are best), and leftover food (mould can grow on food overnight!)
- *all refined carbohydrates* – white flour, white rice, white floured pasta and anything not made from whole grains
- *all stimulants* – coffee and tea, even decaffeinated
- *all smoked or cured foods* – smoked or cured fish, ham, bacon and any other meat.

Looking at the list above, you must now be thinking, 'So what *can* I eat?' The list is just as long.

Foods you can eat

The major foods you can eat are:

- *yeast-free breads* – soda bread, chapatis
- *meat, poultry, and fish* – it is best to buy organic, though, because most meat today contains antibiotics and hormones that are no good for anyone with an already weak immune system (especially for women, eating meat or fish that contains hormones can contribute to dramatic hormonal swings in your body), but if you absolutely cannot eat organic, non-organic lamb and rabbit are safer meats to eat because they are not mass produced, so they are less likely to be given lots of hormones and antibiotics
- *potatoes* – they can be a lifesaver when you go out to eat, but, remember, if you get a jacket potato, ask them to stuff it with

freshly steamed vegetables or something that will not feed the candida – don't smother it with baked beans or cheese!

- *grains* – those that have been processed less are best, so, unfortunately, it would be best to avoid wheat, especially when you are just starting your diet, as it has often been through a lot of processing and often contains mould, but there are other grains, like millet, brown rice, quinoa, spelt and amaranth, that you can eat instead

- *beans and pulses* – great for so many meals – stews, bakes, even burgers (freshly cooked pulses, first soaked overnight, are best to eat, but tinned pulses without added sugar are fine if you are in a rush)

- *unhydrogenated margarines* – any dairy-free, unhydrogenated ones

- *rice cakes, malt-free oatcakes and crispbreads* – make great snacks, just read the ingredients before you buy them so you know exactly what you're eating

- *fresh vegetables* – your body needs fresh vegetables for their nutrients, so steam them, make a soup or stew and discover all the many ways there are to enjoy fresh vegetables, but avoid tinned vegetables as they usually come with sugar and preservatives – get into the habit of buying your vegetables fresh, organic if you can, and eating salads daily

- *herbal tea, mineral water and vegetable juice* – discover the joy of juicing vegetables as it's an enjoyable way to get lots of nutrients into your diet and try hot water on its own or with a bit of lemon – remember, your body needs water (not just any liquid, it should be water) to aid in the release of toxins, so drink six to eight glasses of filtered water per day

- *flours* – any flour but white, processed flours are OK, but try to stay away from wheat at least at the beginning of your diet because of the mould and experiment with other grain-based flours like brown rice, soya or millet flour (if you want to eat pasta, look for pasta made with wheat-free flour – there are many available in healthfood shops)

- *alternatives to cow's milk* – soya milk, oat milk, rice milk and nut milks are very nice and try goat, sheep or soya cheese

- *foods that have antifungal effects* – garlic, leeks, chives and onions are all wonderful foods to eat in abundance on a candida diet because they kill off fungi, moulds and viruses, but not friendly bacteria (you can prevent the smell of garlic on your breath by eating a few sprigs of fresh parsley with the garlic).

Beginning to add these foods into your diet might seem overwhelming at first. 'How am I ever going to substitute soya milk for cow's milk, herbal tea or, even worse, hot water for coffee?' Chapters 4 and 5 will introduce you to some of these new foods and give you helpful hints on how to make the transition to this new diet. Don't worry, many people have done it!

The problem with sugar

Sugar. We love it. Many of us think we can't live without it. Well, you have to. Candida *loves* sugar – it could eat sugar all day and night. Most likely, candida and the sugar you eat have been having a party in your system for a long time. When you stop eating sugar, though, the party will end.

Here are some facts about sugar. The word 'sugar' has two meanings. The first is the more popular definition of sugar, the sweet white or brown sugar spooned into tea or used to make biscuits and cakes. The second meaning is chemical: the sweet tasting, crystalline carbohydrates that are part of many foods we eat like maltose (sugar derived from malted grain), fructose (from fruit) and lactose (from milk). Usually, any ingredient ending in 'tose' means it is a form of sugar. This is important to remember when you are shopping. You must read the ingredients of everything you buy because *sugar hides everywhere*.

Sugar depresses the immune system. When you eat sugar, it goes into your body and begins to metabolize. To do this, it must take what nutrients it is missing from other sources in your body. This means taking from your reserve of nutrients – mostly B vitamins, calcium, phosphorus and iron. Everybody has a different limit to how many nutrients can be depleted from their body before they become nutritionally deficient and sick, but you can be sure that if you eat a lot of sugar, your immune system has to work harder to stay healthy. You can also be sure that the candida in your body is feeding off this sugar and multiplying, making you feel rotten. Every person's body is different, so it is pointless to try and figure out how much sugar it will take before you, your family or your friends get to the point of feeling bad. Better to eliminate sugar from your diet and eliminate candida's food source.

The problems with dairy products

I used to be an ice-cream addict. A tub of Häagen Das, a large spoon and some evenings that would be my supper. I never thought I could give it up, never, but I managed to make it through a year dairy-free. To reward myself, I ate a tub of Häagen Das coffee ice-cream. I felt human again (not to mention a little sick). The second year seemed less difficult, mainly because my body now felt stronger than it had in previous years and the multitude of health problems that had plagued me had virtually disappeared. Could dairy products have been a major culprit?

We have been brought up to believe that eating a lot of dairy products is good for us, will give us strong bones and is just plain healthy. For most people, and candida sufferers in particular, too many dairy products are making our bodies feel sluggish and our immune systems weak. How?

Imagine a meal of cheese, a cream sauce and ice-cream going through the digestive process in your body. All of these are thick and dense, so when they meet the various organs in the digestive system in large quantities, they have a hard time getting through and, like a sieve after you have pressed fruit through it, the pores get clogged. If you eat quite a lot of dairy products on a daily basis, your organs cannot handle the overload, so the excretion processes will not function properly. The result might be that you excrete the excess waste from other areas of your body, like your skin (you may have acne) or it stays in your body, building up and often forming mucus or pus, which is a perfect medium in which bacteria can grow. Candida thrives on undigested milk for just this reason: the mouldy, bacteria-filled environment of the mucus is a comfortable place for it to grow.

Dairy products also produce the perfect environment for other infections to develop. It is not surprising that with the high consumption of dairy products so many common health problems today have to do with the body trying to cope with the build-up and excretion of toxins in the body: asthma, allergies, acne, pimples, obesity, to name just a few. Dairy products are certainly not always the *only* cause of excess build-up of toxins, but they are a large contributing factor and must be considered if someone eats a lot of dairy products and is frequently experiencing ill health.

A FEW MORE FACTS ABOUT DAIRY PRODUCTS

Women tend to suffer more from the build-up of dairy products than men, and it takes longer for them to get such build-ups out of their systems. The link between high consumption of dairy products by women and diseases like breast cancer and gynaeco-logical problems is well documented. I know when I cut out dairy products the cysts on my ovaries that I had suffered from chronically for years disappeared and my periods began coming monthly for the first time in my life. Many allergy specialists now tell people who consume a lot of dairy products and are sick all the time to cut them out of their diet and see how they feel. Often the difference is remarkable.

On the candida diet you can eat goat's and sheep's milk, but not cow's milk. This is because cow's milk is the most difficult to digest. It is mass produced and, as a result, often contains drug residues that an already sluggish body does not want in the system.

Allergies and food intolerances

For candida sufferers, knowing exactly what to eat is often complicated by allergies and food intolerances. You must be aware of these because you could change to a candida diet and still feel bad.

Almost every person with candida will suffer from an allergy or intolerance of at least one food; often they are allergic to many. This is because the candida weakens the immune system, so any excess load is unwelcome. You may get a headache, stomach ache, a rash – allergic reactions come in many forms. An allergic reaction is your body's way of telling you, 'No, I don't want this (food, environment) right now'.

How you tell an allergy from an intolerance

It is generally agreed by traditional allergists and other practitioners who test for allergies that an *allergy* is the immune system's response to a foreign substance. If you are allergic to a particular food, the body's immune system will go on alert, produce antibodies and an adverse reaction will occur.

This is about all that the medical establishment and other allergy practitioners agree on. Views on allergies are wide ranging, some specialists claiming that allergies do not cause severe medical problems, while others insist that allergies are often the culprit behind many of the common health problems that exist today. Candida experts agree with the latter view and feel that you must identify what foods you are allergic to before you begin the candida diet. If not, you could be setting yourself up for disappointment because you will still be eating the wrong foods for you.

A food *intolerance* is similar to an allergy in that it is a reaction someone has to a foreign substance. Intolerances, or 'sensitivities' as some allergists refer to them, are not recognized as readily by the traditional medical establishment as allergies are because they cannot be measured in a scientific way. Despite this, many other natural health practitioners are convinced that food intolerances exist in people whose immune systems are weak. Factors like candida, stress, PMS, and digestive problems can cause intolerances to flare, and then you may only need a small amount of a food to cause a reaction.

In the book *Food Allergies*, the differences between an allergy and an intolerance are summed up in the following way: 'True food allergies are easier to detect, as there is a reaction every time that food is eaten. Food intolerances are like shifting sands, in the sense that the body may or may not react every time, depending on what else is going on. However, the symptoms are much the same for both and can affect almost any part of the body.'

18

How to know what foods you are allergic to

When you begin your treatment for candida, it is best to see an allergist to help identify what foods you react to. The most common food sensitivities are to:

- wheat
- dairy products
- yeast
- corn
- eggs
- beef
- citrus fruits.

Until you begin to know your body better and go to a practitioner to identify your allergies, there are some self-tests you can do at home.

THE PULSE TEST

Do not eat the foods you want to check for five days before you do this test. On the day you want to do the test, your stomach should be empty. Sit in a comfortable place for 15 minutes and then take your pulse. This is your resting pulse. Then eat one of the foods you are testing and take your pulse after 15 minutes, then again after 30 minutes. (It is best to check a food item in its purest state. For example, to check your tolerance to wheat, eat something with wheat as the only ingredient, like Shredded Wheat.) If your pulse rate increases dramatically (usually, more than ten points) then you may be allergic to that food. If you are allergic, keep away from that food for three more days and then do the test again. If allergic symptoms persist, eliminate that food from your diet for a while.

START A FOOD DIARY

This can be lots of fun and gives you a good idea of what foods you are putting into your body and how they make you feel. Write down everything you eat for one week and the time you eat it. Also write down any physical symptoms you feel and the day and time they occur. At the end of the week, look back at your diary to see if there is any correlation between the food you ate and how you felt. If you suspect one or more foods are giving you problems, eliminate them and see how you feel.

One of the major drawbacks of this test is that often, if you eat out, you do not know what ingredients are in your food, so it may be difficult to identify your problem foods. Also, sometimes you may have delayed reactions to foods – the reaction occurring even several days later.

You need to be aware of these drawbacks, but don't let them prevent you from trying this test – many people do identify food allergies this way.

ELIMINATION DIET

For one week, do not eat all the common foods to which you think you are sensitive. If your symptoms subside, continue on the diet for one more week, then begin to add back the eliminated foods, only one per day. Be careful not to add an eliminated food in a form that contains another one of your eliminated foods. For example, if you are eliminating wheat and eggs, don't eat something with wheat that also contains eggs because then you cannot be sure which one you are reacting to. If symptoms do occur after you have reintroduced a food, you probably should avoid that food for a while. To be sure, recheck the food by eating it at five-day intervals to make sure it was not a coincidence that you developed symptoms after eating it.

If your symptoms are not alleviated at all by an elimination diet, then it is possible you are not allergic to the foods you eliminated and you should consider eliminating other foods or look at environmental factors in your life, such as dust, cooking gas or household chemicals, which commonly cause problems for candida sufferers.

The elimination diet can be done by yourself, but people who know they have serious allergic reactions, like asthmatics and small children, are advised to test foods in this way only under the supervision of an allergy specialist.

Don't take drugs Never treat an allergic reaction with drugs without first trying to cure it by eliminating different foods. It just makes no sense, especially if you have candida, because drugs also feed the candida and treat only the symptoms, not the cause of your reaction. If you want to treat the cause, begin to identify what foods produce your ill feelings and eliminate those foods from your diet. Most people feel remarkably better when they do this.

Detoxing: the effect eliminating particular foods can have on your body When you eliminate certain foods from your diet, your body will experience a die-off reaction because the candida has nothing to feed on any more. Also, because the foods you are allergic to have built up in your system and no more of them are entering it, they begin to break down and find their way out of the body. Initially you may feel worse before you feel better, but do not be scared or put off by an increase in symptoms as it means that your body is getting rid of all the stuff that has been causing the problems. Indeed, Michio Kushi, a leader of the macrobiotic movement (dedicated to healthy spiritual and vegan living), describes detoxing as the body's way of 'house cleaning'. He says any of the following symptoms can be experienced when your body detoxes:

- general fatigue
- pains and aches
- fever, chills, coughs
- abnormal sweating and frequent urination
- skin discharges and unusual body odours
- diarrhoea and constipation
- temporary decrease in sexual vitality and desire
- temporary cessation of menstruation
- irritability
- minor transitory symptoms, such as a little hair loss, restless dreams, feeling cold.

Only some of these symptoms will be experienced by most people who are detoxing, depending on how bad your candida and food allergies are. The more your body has to clean out, though, the stronger and longer will be the reaction to your body discharging it. Everyone detoxes at different rates, so comparing yours with another person's is pointless.

Do not discontinue your diet because of detoxification symptoms (see the Food elimination and symptom chart at the back of this book as a handy reference). Friends and family may say, 'Why are you on that diet if it makes you so sick?' Tell them, you're on it because you are actually getting better! Once you go through the detoxification period, most people do feel a lot better. It's like coming out of a dark tunnel into sunlight.

Listening to your inner guide to know what to eat

We all know what we should eat, yet rarely do we listen to our bodies. Having regular 'conversations' with your body is an excellent way to be able to guage what food is right for you. This may initially sound silly. 'How can I talk to my body?', you may say.

Annemarie Colbin suggests doing the following. Relax for a few minutes with your eyes closed. Send a message down to your body, just like you were beaming a sonic wave to the bottom of the ocean. Ask yourself, 'Is this (pick a food) good for me?' A distinct feeling will well up. 'Yes', it's OK, or 'no', it's wrong. Go with your gut feeling.

Colbin stresses one crucial thing to keep in mind while doing this exercise. 'OK' feelings about food are not to be confused with 'delicious'. Ice-cream may be 'delicious', but it will not evoke an 'OK' feeling. Don't forget this advice when you practise this exercise.

Our bodies are constantly giving us 'yes'/'no' signals, telling us what we really want to eat. As you become more in tune with your body, you should instinctively know when to reintroduce foods into your diet.

3

Case histories

A new diet will change your life. There is no doubt about it. The stories that follow take you through some of the highs and lows to expect when you go on a candida diet. As you read them, remember that everyone's body has different needs. What is the right road to recovery for one person may not be the right road for you. Even if what works for you is different to what works for other candida sufferers, the stories in this chapter show you are not alone in your quest to regain your health by changing your diet. Many people have done it and got rid of their candida.

'My family thought I was mad'

Sarah had rheumatoid arthritis for years and decided in 1991 to get help because she did not want to continue taking medication to control her arthritis forever. She saw a friend get a lot better after cutting out foods from her diet, so she decided to go to that friend's health practitioner. When she was told she had candida she was flabbergasted.

To be honest, I didn't really think food was as important as I do now. I mean, you eat things and sometimes after you might think, 'Oh, I didn't like that' or 'I feel a bit sick', but I still used to eat them. It never registered, *don't eat these things*.

When I was handed the sheet of paper telling me what to eat on this candida diet it was frightening. I thought, 'I'm not going to be able to eat anything'. And things I liked I couldn't eat. I always used to love coffee. In the morning, a cup of coffee – oh! – I wouldn't dream of getting up and doing anything without the kettle on and a cup of coffee there. When I saw 'no coffee' on the diet I thought, 'I'm not going to be able to do this. It's rubbish. It can't be right, people have drunk coffee for years'. I did do it, but it was very, very hard. But I thought I wasn't going to lose anything by giving it a go.

Having a family, it was difficult because you've still got to buy things that *you* can't have, but they *can*. Like gravy. I use to love gravy. I hated a dinner if there wasn't a nice gravy. A lovely gravy finishes the dinner – so that was hard, when you're having your dinner dry. Sometimes I poured cauliflower or cabbage water over the dinner, but I like my meal to look colourful and it looked awful. The taste wasn't too bad, though. All along I was telling myself, 'It's nice, I am going to like this', because I didn't want to ache. And now, I don't even think of having gravy.

My family all thought I was mad. They would say to me, 'What are you doing that for? Why don't you eat this?!' I got no support whatsoever. I sometimes thought at first I was mad. Because for years and years people have had these foods and then someone all of a sudden is telling you not to eat them.

If I cheated – and many times in the beginning I did cheat – my kids use to say, 'Oh, you're having a biscuit! You can't do it!' And I think they got pleasure out of saying that. It is hard, and after a while you think, 'Oh, I must be all right now. I could just have that biscuit'. Especially during my period, my taste-buds go crazy and sometimes I'm up against the cupboard thinking, 'No, don't do it!' The next thing, I'd be opening the cupboard again thinking, 'What are you doing?!' Everybody's different with cheating. One of my friends with candida is brilliant. She is a saint. But me, I found it hard not to cheat, especially at first.

When I'd go home to my Mum's house I used to take all my own foods with me and not eat their food. My Mum, she thought I was mad as well. My family's reaction was, 'Oh, we don't think it'll do you any harm. I've been eating that for years and there's nothing wrong with me'. So you get to the point after a while where you tend to keep quiet about it with certain people. But my friends were brilliant about my new diet. At Christmas or at parties, they'd just do me a jacket potato in the oven. It was fine, and they were really good about it.

At work I used to take food with me. The diet is really just about altering your patterns a bit and preparing something to take with you. Usually you'd just get something at work – a sandwich or something – but now you have to give yourself time to prepare something. Once you've done it, it's nothing really. Just altering your patterns. Now I do it, and I just do it. The same with food shopping. You have to look to see what's in things. Like tomatoes, I'm allergic to tomatoes. There are so many things with tomatoes in them. In the beginning you think there is nothing you can eat, but it's amazing how you find alternatives.

Going out was difficult because you don't always know all the ingredients in the meal. Now I do go out, but I choose something plain that I know I can eat. Jacket potatoes are my favourite.

When you start the diet it's like going into a jungle and you don't ever think you're going to get out. After six months I did start to feel a lot better. And now it's become a way of life for me. I feel I've got *go* in me. When before I use to just trudge on, now I can jump! Unless I start eating a lot of biscuits and sweets, I feel good all the time – and I'm off my arthritis medication!

'I always have a "safe meal" ready'

By 1989, Emma felt like she was at death's door. Always sick as a child, it was after her second child in 1987 that her physical health began to deteriorate rapidly. First, she was on antibiotics for acne for 6 months and then she developed a pelvic infection from a fitted coil, for which she took antibiotics for another 18 months. She had frustrating encounters with her doctor, who told her that she had irritable bowel syndrome and then, when her symptoms did not clear up on the high-fibre diet she was put on, that she had a social phobia and needed to go on a ten-week course to relax.

Despite the course, which she felt was useful, her symptoms still persisted until she went to see a nutritionist. He immediately spotted she was a coeliac, so she had a test done at hospital and it confirmed this diagnosis. Yet, on a gluten-free diet and cutting out all the foods she was allergic to, she still did not fully recover. The nutritionist, recognizing how much she gravitated to sugary products, then diagnosed candida.

I was just craving sweet things all the time. One of the things I was told to do when I was just diagnosed as a coeliac was to get up in the morning and have a cup of boiled water before breakfast with a drop of honey in it. Well, I was having honey with a drop of boiled water! When I called up the nutritionist, he suspected candida and said to cut out all the sugar immediately.

It was very hit and miss for me with the diet. He gave you a set of instructions to follow, but of course we're all different and we all react differently, so I really had to find my own way. I was very lucky because my friend had only just been diagnosed with candida a month before me so we were very much in this together and had each other. I don't think I could have done it without her.

I don't think I *had* an immune system at that time. Bombarding my body with too many supplements and too many different foods was too much, so I had to do it very, very gradually. I went through terrible withdrawal for a few weeks. Awful, awful. I thought I was dying. I thought, this isn't right. Every day I'd ring my nutritionist to see if my symptoms were OK. With all the toxins all of a sudden shifting and moving about and the candida dying off as well, I think it's just quite a lot for your body to take.

The diet stayed all the time – I never went off the diet for two to three years. I was so ill, I *couldn't* cheat. Cheating was not an option to me. It wasn't a great problem cooking for the family. I cooked a meal that I could eat and then if my husband wanted to add his oven chips or some cheese, well then that was fine.

My husband believed totally in what was going on in my body. He was a great support – without him I wouldn't have survived. He knew when every doctor was saying – and sometimes when I was thinking – it's in my mind, it wasn't. He was as relieved when I was diagnosed with candida as I was. He was crying as well because he was just so pleased that someone could help me because I think he thought that was it, I was going to die.

I now had a label. When you feel so bad, you're desperately looking for a label, so you can say to people 'I have this'. At work, I was lucky and did not have to explain to anybody that I had candida because I was also a coeliac, and people accept that and they're very concerned and worried about you then. But when you have this candida problem, I think it's a lot harder to explain to people. People are a lot less likely to take it on board – especially people who have no problems at all, they don't understand. I don't think anybody who hasn't had candida does understand. I don't think they can. You get to the stage where people offer you things you can't eat and you say 'No thank you' and they say, 'Oh, well a bit can't hurt you!' And you think, no way, I couldn't even consider trying that little bit. So it is very hard and there's a great stigma attached to it because eating is such a social thing and you're almost a social outcast if you don't eat what everyone else is eating.

Once I was on the diet I decided to tell most people I knew well that I was on it. Everybody then knew and people came to me and began to ask *me* for advice. 'What do you mean, you have food allergies? What happens?' If they wanted to know, I would tell them. And then they would always say, 'Well, *I* get so and so, and so and so – or, my kids have such and such, and such and such'. It went along the grapevine very quickly. You get asked so many questions, you become a nutritionist yourself!

I always made my food at home. If I went out, then I would take a pot of tuna and some rice cakes, because I lived on rice cakes in those days. Also, salads at lunchtime. It was very difficult to know what to eat initially because one week I would get a reaction to say, chicken, and another week I wouldn't. One thing that helped was I always bought my food at the same one or two shops. Then I knew what I was getting every time.

The first time I walked into a healthfood shop I was relieved because I knew that was what I needed. I knew that this was it, this was what I had been waiting for. I was home. I knew this

27

was my last chance to get well and that these new foods would help, because I always knew my ill health was food-related. I felt it in my body and I think we all really know our bodies anyway, but I didn't really know how to do anything about it.

The first year on the diet was hell. It was very up and down and I did not feel in control. I didn't know what was happening to me. But by the end of the first year I began to feel in control. I knew what was happening to me and I knew that if I ate something, what the result would be and I knew how to handle it and how to get better. After the withdrawal stage, when I was ill, my symptoms were never as bad as they were at the very beginning. Sometimes when I did feel bad I had to stop and think, now is this as bad as I used to be? Because when you're really ill like that, when you then become ill in the future you think you're bad again, but until you think about it you realize, 'My God, I am not really *that* bad'.

I always had a 'safe meal'. My safe meal was basmati brown rice, lightly fried up in sunflower oil with a can of tuna. I also cooked peas in with the rice and beansprouts. So, it was sort of my exotic Chinese meal. At the very end I'd grate carrot, so that would give it a bit of colour. So it looked good, it looked appetizing and it was safe. I was OK on that. So, if I had been ill I would always go to my safe meal and I'd be all right. I also used it when my family got a take-away, I'd make this meal and feel OK about not eating their meal. Now I don't even *want* their meal. No way!

Eating the candida diet was worth every bit of struggle because I am now well. I can only explain it as I was dying and now I'm alive.

'I was allergic to everything'

Nine years ago, 43-year-old Louise, despite eating huge amounts of food, was so thin her doctor decided it was due to her gallbladder, so she had it removed. A few months later, still unusually thin, her doctor was not able to explain what was wrong with her. Then a friend of a friend recommended that she see a clinical ecologist. Willing to do anything, Louise went to see him.

He immediately tested me for food allergies and I was allergic to all citrus fruits, dairy products, sugar and chocolate. It was funny because I had already cut out tea and coffee because I knew they were bad for me, so, instead, I was drinking only citrus juice. No wonder I was feeling so bad!

Initially, he did not know I had candida, but he told me to eliminate the foods I tested allergic to. I did and felt better for the first five days. But then the malaise came back across my eyes and all I wanted to do was put my head down. For six weeks it continued and I felt like I was going crazy. I would walk down the supermarket aisle and want to buy anything that had sugar in it.

So, I went back to him and this time he tested me for yeast. He put Marmite under my tongue and then did muscle testing to see if I had candida. Well, I did. Back then, not much was known about candida, but he did give me a diet sheet so I knew what I could and could not eat.

The diet was very, very difficult at first, but I was so sick I would try anything. I never cheated – it just wasn't worth it to me. But, when you are sick, you lose your confidence, so I became a totally different person at work. People thought I was a very withdrawn person when, in fact, just the opposite had always been true! I never ate at work – I would just drink hot water. I only ate at home.

My husband was a tower of strength to me. He ate a lot of my new foods with me, but would still have his puddings. This was crucial in my recovery. I was living on only about five foods in my diet for many years because it ended up I was allergic to everything. All flours, all cooked root vegetables, all nuts and seeds . . . There was practically nothing I could snack on, but I felt so much better when I did not eat these foods it has been worth it.

I now laugh at how uncomfortable it makes people feel when I go for tea and order hot water. The other day this happened with my Mum. We went for tea and she wanted me to order anything *but* hot water, but what I wanted was hot water! It makes me feel good. When I first started on this diet, I had a difficult time asking for hot water. I always offered to pay for it, not wanting them to think I was a down and out trying to get a handout. But now I've realized that if I *want* hot water it's OK. So, I just order it, like it's nothing different to a tea.

How has being on a candida diet changed my life? Well, next week my husband and I are off to Portugal for a holiday. We go on a self-catering holiday so I can make the foods I want. Nine years ago, I rarely left my house. I also never have to go to doctors because I never get sick much. And my weight is finally normal. My doctor cannot believe it when he sees me in the street!

'I just wanted to eat what everybody else was eating'

Throughout childhood, Phil was always getting sick with colds and sinus infections. By his teenage years, he was taking antibiotics regularly. His tonsils were removed when he was 15, which provided some relief, but at 19 he began to work in a factory and experienced severe headaches, fatigue and irritable bowel syndrome. His doctor gave him medication and some dietary advice, but nothing seemed to work.

I was feeling worse and worse. You know, every day just to get out of bed was difficult – an effort. I didn't know what to do any more. My doctor didn't know what to do with me. Luckily my wife's friend suggested I go see her nutritionist.

She got me tested for allergies. I was allergic to everything. Unbelievable, I thought. No way – can't be – but then, after I got some more information from the nutritionist, I thought again and it did make sense. I must have had allergies my whole life.

When I was handed the candida diet sheet I thought it was ridiculous. How was I ever going to eat like that? Impossible. I went home and showed my wife the diet and she also thought it just wouldn't be possible. My wife and I just sat in the lounge and looked at each other in amazement for a while. But then we decided, if this diet was what it was going to take to make me feel better, then I'd better give it a try.

Where I work, everyone brings a packed lunch and we eat together. At lunchtime every day I ate a sandwich. Every day. *Everyone* eats a sandwich. Also, if you don't eat with people, then they'll start talking. I felt really foolish the first day I brought my lunch on the candida diet. My wife made me a baked potato the night before and so I took that and a tin of tuna. When it was lunchtime, I wanted to say I wasn't hungry, but everyone knows how much I usually eat so that wouldn't work. So, I ate my tin of tuna and potatoes. Yeah, everyone laughed at first. They laughed for a while. In the evening, I'd go home and say to my wife, 'I just want to eat what everyone else is eating'. She was really helpful and gave me encouragement to continue – I wouldn't have been able to do it without her.

The other hard habit to change was going for a pint of beer after work or on the weekends. I loved having my pint. At first I couldn't face going to the pub with friends after work. How could I go and *not* have a pint? I always said I was busy after work. Some people made a comment, but I didn't care because I just couldn't face it. Going into a pub and not drinking alcohol seemed crazy to me. Now I do go into pubs and have no problem ordering a soda water. When I started feeling better from this diet, I became less concerned about eating and drinking foods that were different to those of other people.

I can't believe how much energy I have now. And my relationship with my wife has improved a lot because when I felt bad all the time, I couldn't be nice. I'm like a different person now, and all because I was eating the wrong foods for my body before. Imagine that.

'Cheating is a vicious circle'

Six years ago, Katie felt sluggish and always got pains in her knees and legs. She took the Pill for ten years and had had gynaecological problems throughout her adult years. She remembers that as a child she was always fussy about food. She used to take notes to school that said, 'Katie does not like this. Don't give her this in her school dinner'.

I've always had an open mind and believed that a lot of the illnesses around are from the foods we eat. When I was given the candida diet sheet, at first I thought, 'I can't do it', but I'd paid the money to go and see this allergist, so I thought, 'I have to give it a go'.

I changed my diet literally the day after I saw the allergist. In the beginning, I felt a bit tearful – I didn't understand I was going through withdrawal. I found with the least little thing I was crying, it was like I lost my confidence, which wasn't like me. My husband didn't understand it, but was very easygoing about changing his diet. He said, 'Well, that's fine by me, then I'll have what you're having', so he has more or less changed over. He will eat a bit different from me, but mostly we now eat what I call 'wholesome food'.

It has not been easy sticking to the diet. Last week I had a couple of bad days because I cheated. I bought a bun and I ate some chocolate and I feel terrible. I'm just starting to get back into the diet. I seem to go down at Christmas time – I have no willpower. I start eating a few sweets and then it's like a vicious circle. It's easy to start feeling poorly again and then it's harder to get off those foods. And I know sometimes when I'm eating the foods that are bad for me that I'm going to be ill tomorrow, but I can't stop myself.

Last summer I went back to my allergist and I told him I didn't feel good and that I was cheating and he said, 'Look, you're wasting your money coming here because you have got to do it yourself'. So I went home and thought, 'Well, yes, I am stupid'. I had gone for a few months and didn't cheat, but chocolate is my worst thing. And as soon as Christmas comes, you know, you're bringing sweets for other people and then you think, 'I'll just have *one*. One won't hurt me'. But, of course, one leads to two and so on.

When I was very, very strict on the diet, I could get up and climb mountains. There's no doubt about it, the diet does work. In the beginning I use to look at every packet, but now I've got used to it. You also learn what foods you need to cut out and how it changes. Now I've cut out cornflakes because, funnily enough, since I was all right on soya milk, I was also told I could have a few cornflakes. Well, I was eating four or five bowls a day and, in the end, when I got tested for allergies again, I was sensitive to soya and cornflakes.

My friends thought I'd gone a bit loopy in the head when I first went on the diet. So did my sister, but she is always at the doctor – always. A week does not go by without her visiting the doctor. The pain goes from one place to another. First the pain is in her shoulder, then it's in her neck. And I've tried to tell her – she knows she's allergic to so many foods, but she eats everything. And so she tells me I get on her nerves, me and my food. I don't really take any notice of it because I know that I'm healthier than she is. Her food is her comfort in life. I think for many of us it is that way, but it has to change.

If I go out for a meal, I will ring the restaurant up beforehand and order a separate meal. People at restaurants don't mind that, they are geared to it – especially with lots of vegetarians around now – and they are pretty good. At first, I felt uncomfortable about asking for a special meal. We would go from one restaurant to the other. I'd look at the menu and say, 'Oh, no, I've got to leave here – there's nothing I can eat' and so rather than ask them to do something special, I would just leave, but now I don't care, I just ask them.

I have had people over to eat and cooked my foods. When they say, 'What's this?', I say it's minced beef and they don't know it's minced soya. Then, after they've eaten it, I tell them it's soya and they can't believe it didn't taste any different. If I make people a sandwich and they say they'd like butter, I use unhydrogenated soya margarine and they don't know the difference.

Now I listen to other ladies my age, and they're on this tablet and that tablet, and I feel healthy. I *am* healthy. I haven't had to go to the doctor for years. I take no medication. It is expensive trying to get better, taking all the supplements, but I decided to spend my money on getting better. You've got to think, 'quality of life' – that's how I look at it.

Hopefully these stories have motivated you to start your candida diet soon. You *can* feel better. Each story in this chapter demonstrates this. The next chapter will help you get started on your road to recovery.

4

Getting started on your diet

*'The intelligence of our bodies knows what is good for it.
Once that intelligence is channelled through correct habits
– and this involves making conscious decisions at the
beginning – then eating problems and risks of a wrong diet
disappear'.*

Deepak Chopra, *Creating Health*

When I was first diagnosed with candida, I was convinced this new
diet would never fit into my lifestyle. I was in shock. Luckily my
kinesiologist told me to 'Go buy a cookbook'. This was just what I
needed to do – if I was going to get better, I had to get started on the
diet.

You too have to get started on the diet. Letting yourself believe
'I can't cook', 'I have no time to cook' or 'there will be nothing to
eat when I go out to a restaurant' is self-defeating. If you continue
to think this way, you will not succeed on this diet. The people who
have had the most success are the ones who began the diet thinking
positively and were willing to experiment with new ideas. A
positive attitude makes for a positive outcome.

Below are a few ways you can make a positive start to a candida
diet.

- *Make a commitment* The sooner you get on the diet, the quicker
  you will recover. Many candida sufferers ask, 'Will I ever be
  able to eat ''normal'' food again?' (Ironically, most people who
  have been on a candida diet now think processed, sugary foods
  are 'abnormal'!) This diet does not have to be a lifelong
  commitment, but it does have to be for as long as it takes you to
  feel better.
- *Take a wholefood cookery class* This is an excellent way to feel
  more comfortable cooking all your new foods. Ask around if
  anyone in your area cooks wholefoods or put an ad in your local

paper. You may be surprised to find that one of your neighbours is a wholefood cook or knows one! Ask your local Council if it would be willing to sponsor someone to come and give a cooking class or series of classes on cooking for special diets (see the Useful addresses section at the back of this book).

- *Read, study and ask questions about candida and the diet* Books on candida are available, but also read books on topics related to healing and special diet cookbooks. Ask someone at your local healthfood shop for a book recommendation or if they know someone in the area who could teach you more. Remember, a lot of health-orientated people walk into healthfood shops, so yours could be full of information – if you ask!

- *Start where you are* Only you know what factors make this diet easy or hard for you to stick to. Take into account what your lifestyle is like. Are you a single mother with small kids? A newly married couple with a hectic work and social life? All of these factors must weigh heavily when you design your candida diet.

Four steps to creating a meal plan that works for you

Once you have made the commitment to change your food habits and try new things, creating a candida meal plan can be fun and enjoyable. You may think, 'I don't need a meal plan, I'll just start'. That is OK if that's what feels right for you, but many people find it helpful to have a plan for at least the first month of the diet. A plan takes the panic out of your mind when you return home from a long day and cannot think of anything to eat. If you take 30 minutes at the beginning of the month to plan your meals, then you don't have to waste precious energy and worry the rest of the month figuring out what to eat.

A meal plan does not mean you are locked into a routine. On the contrary, a meal plan assists you in breaking free from eating routines. Below is a four-step process for creating a candida meal plan. It is easy to follow and can get you on your way to eating a candida diet.

To create your own meal plan you will need:

- a quiet, relaxing space where you can think without interruption for 30 minutes
- a pencil (with an eraser) and a coloured pen
- A4 paper or several large index cards
- a list of the candida diet guidelines (see Chapter 2 of this book)
- a list of the foods you are allergic to or suspect you may be allergic to (it is best to have been tested for food allergies so you know for sure what foods you react to).

Step 1: Consider all your lifestyle factors

Answer the following questions on one index card or an A4 sheet of paper. Put the heading 'Lifestyle factors' at the top of the page.
- How often do I eat at home? At work? Go out to eat?
- How much time do I have to prepare meals?
- Would the people I live with be willing to go on this diet with me and provide support?
- What three things are causing me the most stress in my life at this moment?

Step 2: Pick foods you want to eat

Look at the list of foods permitted on a candida diet (pages 13–15) and the list of your food allergies. Make a list of all the foods you *want* to eat that you are *not* allergic to. Also write down foods you may have never tasted, but are willing to try.

Put the heading 'Candida foods' at the top of the page. Then, with a coloured pen, indicate next to the food if it is 'G' for 'Grain', 'B' for 'Beans', 'V' for 'Vegetable' or 'M' for 'Meat'. If you are a vegetarian, obviously exclude the meat. If you are a meat eater, you might eat fewer beans. These are the staples in a candida diet. Don't worry right now about any foods that don't fit into these categories.

Step 3: Decide what foods you are going to eat and when

Now you are ready to make your personal candida meal plan. Read through all the instructions in this section before you begin. Then, take out your 'Lifestyle factors' list and your 'Candida foods' list.

On A4 paper, draw lines to resemble a monthly calendar. If you are using index cards, make a weekly calendar, using one card for each week. The first date on the calendar is the day you decide to start. Leave enough space on each day to fit your staple foods – grains, beans, vegetables and meats.

On each day, write in what grains, beans, vegetables and meats you will eat. I suggest working with one category at a time for the whole month, say, decide all the days you'll eat grains that month in one go, then all the days you'll eat beans and so on.

Return to your 'Lifestyle factors' list often to remind yourself of your limits so your plan will be realistic. For example, on the days you know you'll have little time to cook, decide to eat foods that will allow you to make a quick meal, like corn pasta (G) with steamed vegetables (V) and Lemon, Garlic and Oil Dressing. On a day you will be eating out, think of what foods from your list you may be able to get at a restaurant, like a jacket potato. As candida sufferer, Sarah, pointed out in Chapter 3, going on a candida diet is just about 'altering your patterns'.

Always be aware of the importance of rotating your foods, to decrease the chances of you becoming sensitive to more foods, which can happen when you eat too much of one food. To do this, as you fill in foods throughout the month, make sure you're eating them every fourth day, not every day. Again, working with one category at a time makes this easier. For example, if you plan to eat rice on Monday, you can eat rice again Friday, then Tuesday, then Saturday. If the range of foods you have to choose from is very limited because of food allergies, then try to leave a day or two between eating the same foods. You must break out of food ruts! You may be able to eat a particular food today, but if you eat it every day for many weeks, most candida sufferers find that, after a while, they cannot tolerate that food any more.

Step 4: Menu plan for the week

Now that you have decided what staple foods you want to eat, each week you need to spend 15 minutes planning how you are going to put them into your meals.

Look at your staple foods for each day and prepare meals

around those foods. Always include a snack for the day, so you have food in a hurry. And remember to look at your 'Lifestyle factors' sheet to remind you of your limits.

So, if your staples were brown rice (G), carrots (V), kale (V), leeks (V) and organic chicken (M), your menu for that day might look like this.

- *Breakfast* Puffed brown rice and soya milk.
- *Lunch* Carrot soup with brown rice and toasted sesame seeds (if you're taking lunch with you, pack some brown rice cakes and a spread, like hummus, instead of the cooked brown rice and bring the soup with you if you have access to cooking facilities).
- *Dinner* Lemon gingered chicken, brown rice and steamed carrots, kale and a creamy leek sauce.
- *Snack* Toasted sunflower seeds.

Balance and flexibility are key to successful meal planning. When you plan, keep in mind your current state of health, the weather and seasons (that is, plan warming foods, like stews, for winter and cooling foods, like salads, for summer), your individual tastes and, of course, your lifestyle factors.

Helpful hints for preparing meals

Keep meals simple

Preparing fewer foods and eating them in their most natural state is healthier and often more enjoyable than something elaborate. Putting lots of ingredients in sauces and other dishes increases the risk of you reacting to all those ingredients and increases your time in the kitchen. Less is best.

Yeast can hide in your kitchen

Old vegetables often have mould on them, especially if they are organic because they haven't been sprayed with tons of chemicals to retain a *fresh* look. Refrigerating your vegetables can help them keep longer. Nuts, oils and seeds should be refrigerated because they will get mouldy. Wooden cutting boards also carry yeast, so clean them very well, regularly, or use plastic cutting boards.

Leftover food gets mouldy, so it is best to avoid food that has been prepared 24 hours or more beforehand. Most candida sufferers can get away with preparing food the night before and then eating it for lunch the next day, but some cannot. If your condition is severe, you might be best avoiding leftovers altogether for a while.

Make a shopping list

When you are just beginning a candida diet, many of the foods you are going to eat will be new to you. Shopping with a list ensures that you will not forget the foods you need to buy. Use your menu plan to make a shopping list so you know what staples to buy. For vegetables, be flexible – if the ones on your list are not in the shop or are not fresh, don't buy them, pick a different vegetable.

Learn cooking tricks

Cooking tricks can save you a lot of time. Learning cooking tricks comes from reading different cookbooks or going to cookery classes. Here are a few helpful tricks I have learned.

- *Cleaning leeks with ease* Leeks can trap dirt between their layers, so cut the leek in half lengthwise. Hold each half under running water, separating the layers to let the water run through them. When the dirt is out, turn them cut side down to drain.
- *Taking the peel off garlic* Peeling garlic can be quick and easy. Put the garlic on a chopping board. Take a wide-bladed knife, put the garlic under the flat part of the knife and press hard. The garlic skin should loosen so much that it almost falls off.
- *Softening beans and avoiding gas* Soak all beans overnight – even small beans, like lentils. Discard the soaking water and add fresh water. Cook them together with kombu, a sea vegetable you can buy in healthfood shops. You can take the kombu out when you've finished cooking or leave it in and eat it!

Prepare the same basic foods for everyone

If the people you eat with at home are not eating your foods, you can still prepare the basic foods you eat, take out a portion for yourself, then add extra spices, ingredients or sauces for the others. Don't make more work for yourself by trying to prepare completely different meals for you and your family.

Atmosphere is important

What makes a good meal is not always just the food. Flowers, an attractive tablecloth on the dining table, candles and a plate of colourful food are all very satisfying ways to brighten the atmosphere and nourish yourself and everyone else at the table. These 'finishing touches' take surprisingly little time to do, and are worth it.

Digestion or indigestion – how to eat

Millions of people in the UK every day rush around and, when they have a moment, quickly cram food into their mouths. If we're not eating as quickly as we can, then many of us are eating in an anxious emotional state. Sometimes we are conscious of how worked up we are when we eat, but often we are not. The result is indigestion, because proper digestion usually will not occur in a stressed or unhappy person.

Deepak Chopra, well-known health spokesperson on the mind–body link with health, believes that proper digestion will not occur if we continue with self-destructive eating patterns. In his book *Creating Health*, he suggests seven guidelines which will allow your mind and body to join together and help you digest and assimilate food properly, which are:

1. pay attention to eating
2. pause momentarily before eating and sit in silence – or say grace – so that the awareness begins the meal quietly
3. eat when you are hungry, and do not eat when you are not hungry

4. do not sit down to eat if you are upset – your body is better off without food until you feel better
5. take time to eat, chewing well and slowly
6. appreciate the company and compliment the cook (even if it's yourself!)
7. avoid eating in any company that makes you feel less than agreeable, but eat with congenial company, friends and family, when you can.

Write these guidelines down, maybe on an index card so you can carry it around with you or put it on your refrigerator in the kitchen and before you eat, think about them. Maybe adopting every one now is not possible for you. I know number four, 'Do not sit down to eat if you are upset', is a real challenge for candida sufferers because you're always upset if you're feeling sick all over! Introduce one at a time and then, when you're ready, introduce more. Being conscious of how to eat well is the quickest way to good health. And as your mind gets better, so will your digestion.

The well-stocked kitchen

Having the right equipment in your kitchen is essential for a candida diet because you will be preparing fresh food on a daily basis. If you don't have the proper tools to make many of these dishes, then it will be a lot more difficult to prepare the food you need for good health.

Every candida kitchen should have the following:

- *Food processor* This relatively small financial investment will significantly increase your meal repertoire. Soups, porridge, spreads and many more dishes become easy when you have a food processor.
- *Stainless steel or enamel cookware* The pots and pans you cook in are important because whatever they are made of will get into your food and if the cookware is of poor quality, you could feel sick. Do not use aluminium cookware because aluminium is a dangerous chemical in high doses in your body. Studies have

shown that when water is heated in an aluminium pot, the aluminium level in the water increases by 75 per cent. Most tap water is safer than this level. Stainless steel and enamel cookware, though, are safe and worth buying.

- *Good, sharp knives* Chopping vegetables with bad knives or unsharpened knives is a great way to frustrate yourself. One really good large and one good small knife, and you'll feel born again. Keep them sharp, and you will be able to happily chop away.
- *Plastic, air-tight containers and glass jars* Containers and jars of different sizes, good quality and with tight seals, are crucial. You will have so many things to store – grains, leftovers for a day, food you want to freeze. Containers are also excellent for people on the go, for packing a lunch in or a snack. Jars are great for storing grains and pulses. Ask friends and family to keep their leftover jars for you, and soon you will be inundated with free glass jars!
- *Resealable bags* You'll use a lot of these if you work outside the home. They are perfect for snacks and storing food.
- *Brush to clean vegetables* A good brush can make cleaning vegetables practically effortless. I have found that thick-bristled brushes from China work best. Look in your healthfood shop and if they don't have any, ask them if they can get some.
- *Stainless steel steamer* An indispensable, cheap addition to your kitchen. These steamers fit in almost all pots and encourage you to get out of the habit of boiling your vegetables.

Every candida kitchen should think of buying:

- *a juicer* fresh vegetable juices taste wonderful and are full of nutrients
- *ginger grater* a grater makes using ginger easy – you don't need to chop the ginger up finely, just take off the skin and grate (ginger is a miracle spice, it helps nausea and is heat-producing, so most candida sufferers should use a lot of it)
- *rubber spatula* indispensable for getting all the food out of a bowl easily.

Every candida kitchen should never have the following:

- *Microwave* Sorry, I know most people have microwaves these days, but microwaves change the basic energy in food, killing 'live' food which means food that is microwaved will have little or no nutritional value. No definitive studies have been able to prove microwaves change the molecular structure of all foods in a bad way, but most food experts agree that microwaving food makes the food less nutritious. This includes 'just' defrosting or reheating food in the microwave. The only exception I would make is, if you are not very sick, to allow yourself to use a microwave once in a while when you take food to work where a microwave is the only way to reheat your food. For some candida sufferers who are very sensitive to their environment, though, just having a microwave in their kitchen (that other people in the family use) could cause them to feel sick. If you must have a microwave for other people to use, put it in a room you do not use very much.

How to have fun with your new foods

Have a candida dinner party

Imagine your family or friends' responses to being served some of the foods on your candida diet. The more unusual the food, the funnier the response. I like serving sea vegetables (like hiziki, nori or arame, available at most healthfood shops). Faces wrinkle when you tell them what it is and eyebrows lift way up high when they pick up their fork to eat it. The picture is priceless.

You may think it's a bold move to have a candida dinner party – 'How could I serve someone sea vegetables?' – but introducing your new foods to friends and family by allowing them to try them is usually a great way to make you and them more comfortable about your new diet. People may laugh at the food, but they are usually laughing only because they don't understand this way of eating. It's all new to them (and you!), so, demystify healthy eating for them!

Before the meal, learn a few interesting bits of information about the food you're serving, like the nutritional benefits of sea vegetables. Write this information in different colours on index cards and put the cards on the table before the meal. During the meal, use these cards to explain the foods that are being served and why you need to eat them. Share your mixed feelings about cooking these 'weird' foods and how you first felt making a dish with a new food, like sea vegetables. Invite your dinner guests to share their mixed feelings about eating this food. Allow the conversation to go anywhere. Usually, though, you will have everyone only too eager to express their feelings on food!

You may feel embarrassed and alone at first, but usually by the end of the meal you will feel more dedicated to your healing journey and very proud of yourself for taking a risk. Some recipe suggestions for a candida dinner party are in Chapter 5.

Theme meals

This is a great way to get kids or your partner to try eating candida foods. The foods on a candida diet may initially seem boring and tasteless, but with a little atmosphere and certain food combinations, you can have a meal everyone wants to eat.

Dress up in black and white, put white candles on the table, play some Spanish music and you have 'Mexican night'. Or put on your blue jeans, a baseball cap, rent an American cowboy video and you have 'Yankee night'. Put a blanket on the floor, eat with plastic cutlery and you have 'Picnic night'. Any theme you choose is the right theme. Kids and adults love it. See the menu suggestions in Chapter 5 for the three themes mentioned here.

Find a healing friend

Finding someone you can relate to who also has candida or having a good friend who can empathize with you about your new foods and health needs, is a crucial part of your recovery. Sometimes you just need to brainstorm with someone about how you're feeling and what you need to do about it. A good healing friend does this and also asks you for help. A good healing friend cooks with you and enjoys your cooking. A good healing friend makes you laugh, dance or sing and forget your troubles at just the right time. A good healing friend is that kindred spirit and a whole lot more.

If you cannot think of anyone who fits the 'good healing friend' description, then create your own. Sit quietly, close your eyes and imagine yourself walking through the woods. The path through the woods leads to a small cottage. At the door stands your healing friend. Now open your eyes and write that healing friend a letter, introduce yourself and tell them what you want in the friendship. Later on, make a conscious effort to become this friend to people you meet and soon you will find a healing friend comes into your life. It could be a person you meet at a cookery class or an old friend who you never thought would be perfect for this role. Enjoy their friendship and watch things change.

Eat from a special bowl or plate

If you think your new foods are unexciting, spice them up with a special healing bowl or plate. A bright yellow bowl or a plate with lots of earth tones can be just the right addition to your meal that takes you out of the candida diet blues. When I was feeling my worst with candida, my forest green Chinese-style bowl got me through a lot of sad moments. It represented stability and healing. I could always count on it to pick me up when I was feeling down. I also had an orange plate, to symbolize the healing that needed to take place in my liver.

Learn about what colours are said to heal what parts of your body and then buy a bowl in the colour that heals the area that's out of balance. Alternatively, choose your favourite colour. Buy any style and size of bowl or plate that is right for you. Chinese-style bowls are wonderful because you can eat any meal out of them.

Spend time in a healthfood shop

This should be one of the first things you do when you start the diet. If you've never been to one before you may think 'They're so expensive' or 'I don't know what to buy'. Healthfood shops vary dramatically, but most do have many affordable products (think of all the money you're saving not buying processed foods!) and there are lots of things you can buy in them that are yeast-free, dairy-free and sugar-free. So, the sooner you get to your nearest healthfood shop, the better.

To make the most of your first trip, it is best to plan ahead. What products might you want to buy? If you have no idea, just remind yourself that whatever you buy it must be part of the candida diet, so read the ingredients of every item. There are a lot of unhealthy foods even in healthfood shops. When you walk in, if you feel confident enough, ask to speak to someone working at the shop who could help you identify foods suitable for a candida diet (bring your list of candida foods, because some shopkeepers will not know). This person may also be a good source of information about local cookery classes for special diets or new books on healing.

Once you begin to see the healthfood shop as your friend in healing, eating candida foods will become easier.

Strategies for eating out

You *can* eat out. Of course every candida person is different, and many stop going out for a while when they first go on the diet because eating out seems too difficult on top of all the other hurdles of the diet. If you want (or have) to go out to eat a lot, here are some strategies to ease the panic and make it enjoyable.

- Call the restaurant or host before you arrive and tell them your dietary needs. Most restaurants and all good hosts want to provide food that you can eat. If you call the restaurant on the day you plan to go, about 10 or 11am, and ask to speak to the chef, they will most likely be happy to create a menu using the foods you can eat. I know this was a hard step for me to take, but once I did, the response I got was overwhelmingly positive. At a wedding, I didn't tell the chef in advance about my dietary requirements so I expected to eat nothing, but once I opened my mouth and said I needed special food, the plate of vegetables and rice they made me was the best meal I'd ever had at a wedding. Many people are getting used to catering for special diets, so don't feel shy – just ask!
- Find a favourite restaurant. Think about what restaurants there

are in your area and find at least one that offers one or two dishes you can eat and you enjoy. This is your safety restaurant. When friends or work colleagues want to go out to eat, suggest this restaurant.

- Eat something small before you go. A snack or even a mini-dinner can be a lifesaver if you are going somewhere you think there will be nothing for you to eat. It is better to have something in your stomach, than to sit at the table with an empty stomach and find out the food isn't prepared how you asked.

Learn about the foods you're eating

Going on a candida diet is the perfect opportunity to read books on food and healing. Make time to spend a few afternoons at a bookshop, library or healthfood shop and browse through the books on health, cooking and self-help. Many of these books will answer a lot of your questions about 'why' (why me? why no sugar? why cook?). You also may just meet a 'healing friend' in the health section!

Start a food/mood diary

This is a wonderful way to learn how to listen to your body. You may *think* you're paying attention to everything you eat and how you feel afterwards, but writing it all down and then looking back can put your food and moods in perspective. Here's what to do:

First, find a blank notebook and answer the following questions.

- What were my moods like before candida?
- What moods do I experience now?
- What do I want my moods to be like in five years from now?

Remember, moods can be good and bad.

Then, eat and write down what foods you are eating. Fifteen minutes later, record how you feel. You can write down a word to describe your feeling or draw how you feel. Anything that conveys your mood. If you cannot think of what mood you are in, write anything down, even if it's, 'I cannot think what mood I'm in!'

Be aware that you can have a delayed reaction to some foods, so record *all* mood swings that come throughout the day, even if they do not occur directly after eating.

After one week, look back at your food/mood entries and reflect on the initial three questions you answered. Which mood made you feel like question number 1, number 2 or number 3? Identify the food you ate to create that mood. Begin to eat more of the foods that put you in a better mood. Continue the diary until you feel you don't need or want it any more.

Do the organic carrot experiment

I cannot stress enough the benefits of eating organic food. Foods sprayed with chemicals are not good for us, especially a person with candida who already has an overload of toxins in their immune system. Washing vegetables well or peeling the skin off will not get rid of the chemicals, they are in the cell structures of the vegetables. According to Joanna Blythman in her book *The Food We Eat*, 'a 1994 government spot check on British winter lettuces grown under glass revealed that a quarter of them were contaminated with illegal or excessive levels of pesticides'.

Organic vegetables and meats are not only healthier, but taste better. Not convinced yet? Do the carrot experiment. Buy 1 kg (2¼ lbs) of organic carrots and 1 kg (2¼ lbs) non-organic carrots and wash them well. Take a deep breath and, when you feel relaxed, continue.

- Chop half a non-organic carrot into strips and slowly, with your eyes closed, eat it raw. Record how it tastes, in three words. Then do the same for the organic carrot. Compare your answers.

Not convinced yet?

- Steam an organic and non-organic carrot. Do the same test as above.

Not convinced yet?

- Make a quick carrot soup. Put two large carrots in a saucepan with water. Let them boil for 15–20 minutes. Process the carrots and cooking liquid in your food processor until you have a smooth and soupy mixture. Do this for both the organic and non-organic carrots. Then taste.

It's your choice whether to buy organic or not, but remember that it is not only putting the *right* food into the body that helps a sick person get healthy, it must also be of the best quality.

Enrolling the support of our partner

Most candida practitioners agree that if you have a supportive partner, you will heal quicker and it will be much easier to stay on the diet. A supportive partner accepts your ups and downs and helps you through the process of rebounding to good health. Most partners who are unsupportive are this way because they do not understand what you are going through.

Here's what you can do to enroll the support of your partner. Find a quiet time to sit down with your partner and talk about your feelings on a physical and emotional level. Put on soft, relaxing background music and keep the lights dim. Agree not to answer the phone during your conversation or allow any other interruptions.

Begin by telling your partner how you have been feeling, starting as far back as you can remember 'candida-like' symptoms appearing. If you are getting panic attacks, tell them about these and describe an instance when you had one and how it made you feel. Or describe what it has been like to have pain in your stomach and bloating all the time. Then talk about your new candida diet and your hopes and fears about embarking on such a diet. Tell them what you need and expect of them during your time of healing. Thank them for listening to you.

It is very important to go through this exercise with your partner because your not feeling good affects them too. Neither of you should deny this. A partner can be more understanding, accepting your new diet and even joining you on the diet once they have been told in a calm and loving way how you are feeling. Otherwise, as strange as this may seem, they may not know how you feel.

Meeting the needs of children with candida

If you are a parent trying to get your child on a candida diet, you could feel overwhelmed by the challenge of weaning them off processed foods and sweets. You can be successful in getting them to eat candida foods using patience, humour and actively involving your child. Here are some suggestions.

- Slowly replace processed foods with candida foods. Give them unsugared cereals for sugar-coated ones, soya milk for milk.
- Prepare candida foods that are familiar in appearance. Cook tofu-walnut burgers, baked chips, sweet potatoes.
- Include your child in the preparation of meals. Young children usually love to help. This may seem difficult if your child is older and unaccustomed to helping in the kitchen or you feel you have little time to let them help, but it is very important. Let them grate carrots, wash vegetables or clean beans. Most kids love to eat things they were involved in making.
- Pack popcorn with their lunch, a socially acceptable snack, so they have something to eat when other kids are munching on processed snacks. Of course your child will inevitably eat with other kids, and be tempted by their sweets, but if they have a nutritious snack with them at least they have an option not to eat the sweet.
- Believe that your child can make the switch to candida foods and that their health will greatly improve. If you don't believe it will work, it probably won't. So many children have become healthier and their behaviour, including signs of autism, markedly improved once they went on a candida diet.

Cheating You will not get better if you cheat a lot on this diet. The candida has to die and cannot do so unless you starve it, which means not eating certain foods. Sometimes life circumstances make a new way of eating seem impossible. Respect your limits and know when it is the right time for you to start a candida diet. The sooner, the better, but if you go on the diet and constantly cheat, you only prolong the amount of time you will have to stay on the diet strictly.

Candida sufferers who have been seriously ill for a long time rarely cheat because getting better feels like a matter of life or death for them. If you are not 'deathly sick' you may be more tempted to cheat periodically. 'Oh, this one chocolate bar won't hurt me'. Think again – one chocolate bar could erase all the hard work you put into staying on the diet up until that point.

If you really want a piece of chocolate, go ahead, have it, but eat only half of it and record how you feel afterwards. Once you feel the connection between eating certain foods and feeling bad, you probably won't cheat too many times. If you do not cheat, the candida dies off and cravings for junk food often cease.

Will I ever get off this diet?

The first question most candida sufferers usually ask is, 'Will I ever get off this diet?' and 'When?' We have been conditioned by Western medicine to have an answer and a figure to go with that answer. It's OK to be told, 'You have a bladder infection and it will clear up two weeks after you take this medicine' or 'You have to have a back operation and won't be on your feet for six months to a year'. But when we are told, 'You need to create a diet with foods that suit your body and how long it will take you to feel better depends on you', it leaves so much of the control in our hands, it frightens many of us.

Most people with candida who adhere to the diet strictly and receive proper nutritional treatment are able to come off the diet. The amount of time you will have to stay on the diet, however, depends on your body's needs. If you have been feeling bad for a very long time, you may be on the diet for a couple of years. Others are off, at least the strict portion of the diet, in six months. Being on a candida diet is only one step in your healing process. It is a crucial step, but there are other aspects, discussed in Chapter 6, to feeling better that will determine how fast you get better. Many former candida sufferers find that, over time, their tastes in foods change and they now prefer eating a wholefoods diet, with the occasional sweet, which helps them get well and stay well.

Pressuring yourself to know, 'Will I be on this diet for four months or eight months or a year or three years?' is pointless. You have an exciting opportunity to take control of your own health, so commit yourself to being on a candida diet for however long it takes to feel better.

5

Recipes to please

Every day we need to eat, whether we like it or not. And every day we have to make choices about *what* to eat, whether we like it or not. I cannot stress enough, everyone is different. Candida sufferers, in particular, often have different food sensitivities. If the list of foods you cannot eat seems like it's five miles long right now, don't let that stop you from reading through the recipes in this chapter. You may find that many recipes are OK for you, but even if you don't, reading recipes is a great way to generate ideas about what to cook. You can prepare the same *type* of food, like a 'bake', using a grain, pulse or vegetable you can eat.

The recipes in this chapter use some ingredients you will be familiar with and some you will not. Trying new foods can be an exciting way to make your diet more interesting, so please, do experiment. Aim to cook one dish a week that introduces a new ingredient. You may be amazed at how good new food can be!

All recipes are dairy-free and, of course, sugar-free and yeast-free. Many are also gluten-free. Some people with candida might be able to eat more ingredients than those contained in these recipes. Deciding what ingredients are right for you is best done in consultation with your health practitioner and by taking time every day to assess how your body is reacting and what it is telling you it wants (not what foods are delicious!).

Your exciting adventure into healthy eating is about to begin, so take a deep breath and let's go!

BREAKFAST

You don't have time for breakfast? Set your alarm 15 minutes earlier and *make* time! This is a very important meal in your day, especially if you have low blood sugar, which is very common among candida sufferers. If you are pressed for time, at least sit down and eat a bowl of cereal (home-made muesli or another sugar-free cereal from the healthfood shop) with soya milk or any other non-dairy alternative. Your body will thank you.

The recipes below take between 10 to 20 minutes to prepare. If you put them on to start cooking when you get up, by the time you have showered and dressed, your breakfast will be ready. They really are quick meals.

All the breakfast recipes serve one person.

Porridge

If you use organic oats it tastes a lot better, just like you've added butter!

250 g (9 oz) oats
500 ml (17 fl oz) filtered water

Put the oats and water in a pan and bring to a rapid boil. Turn off the heat, cover and let sit for 10–15 minutes (you can take a shower and get dressed during this time!) Then, eat and enjoy.

Variations
Use soya milk instead of water, for a richer taste.
Add toasted sunflower seeds for more flavour.

Millet and Quinoa Porridge

Millet and quinoa are two wonderful gluten-free grains that you should get to know.

This may sound like a strange combination, but it tastes surprisingly nice and is filling.

120 g (4½ oz) quinoa
120 g (4½ oz) millet
750 ml (1¼ pints) filtered water

Put the millet, quinoa and water in a saucepan and bring to the boil. Turn down the heat and let simmer for 20 minutes. Blend everything together in a food processor until it looks smooth and creamy. Now it's ready.

Variations
Cook with a handful of linseeds.
Millet is a great, creamy porridge in its own right. Boil up 250 g (9 oz) of millet, one carrot and 1 litre (1¾ pints) water. Cook for 20 minutes, puree it and you have a sweet-tasting breakfast porridge.

Sesame and Rice Porridge

If you feel your candida is not too severe, use rice left over from the night before. It will then only take 5 minutes to reheat, instead of 40!

> *200 g (7 oz) brown rice*
> *500 ml (17 fl oz) filtered water*
> *Sesame seeds, to taste*

Bring the rice and water to a boil in a pan, then reduce the heat and simmer for 40 minutes. While the rice is cooking, or the night before, toast the sesame seeds in a dry pan over a high heat, turning them frequently, until they smell toasted. Watch them constantly as they burn easily. Leave them to cool, then store in an airtight jar. When the rice is done, blend until smooth. Add sesame seeds until the flavour is as you like it.

Variations
Use soya milk instead of water for a richer taste.
Add a grated carrot for sweetness.

Muesli

Muesli can be made with any combination of oats, millet flakes, brown rice flakes, barley flakes, nuts and seeds. All of these ingredients can be bought in a healthfood shop. Experimenting with ingredients that you are not sensitive to is the key. Here are a few ideas.

- Combine 450 g (1 lb) oats, 350 g (12 oz) barley flakes, 350 g (12 oz) wheat flakes, 175 g (6 oz) brown rice flakes, a handful of sunflower seeds and coconut flakes.
- For a gluten-free alternative, combine 350 g (12 oz) millet flakes, 175 g (6 oz) brown rice flakes, sesame seeds, and a nut and seed mixture to taste (grind the nuts and seeds up in a coffee grinder).

Scrambled Tofu

This takes 15 minutes to prepare.

1 teaspoon oil   *½ carrot, grated*
½ onion, finely chopped   *½ celery stick, finely chopped*
¼ teaspoon turmeric   *100 g (4 oz) tofu*

Heat the oil in a pan. Sauté the onion and turmeric for 1 minute. Add the vegetables, beginning with the carrot, then the celery. Sauté for 3–5 minutes.
Crumble the tofu into a bowl, then add to the sautéd vegetables and stir. Cover to steam for 5 minutes, stirring occasionally.

Variations
Add some Bragg soy sauce at the end to give it a salty taste. (Bragg is an unfermented soy sauce suitable for people with candida and available at some healthfood shops).
Add ginger or garlic.
Garnish with fresh parsley.

LUNCH

Do you eat lunch out every day? Do you eat at home and tend to eat the same thing? Eating a candida lunch takes a bit of planning in the beginning because your usual patterns will have to change, but once you develop a new routine, eating candida foods at lunchtime becomes a *new* easy pattern.

Baked beans

This can be served over a jacket potato, brown rice, or toasted yeast-free bread.

*200 g (7 oz) dried haricot
  beans*
1 large onion, diced
1 tablespoon olive oil
*5 medium tomatoes,
  quartered*

*2 tablespoons tomato purée
  (make sure it contains no
  citric acid)*
1 teaspoon paprika
freshly ground black pepper

Soak the haricot beans overnight. The next day, drain the beans and cook them for 1 hour in 1 litre (1¾ pints) fresh filtered water until soft.
Sauté the onion in the oil for 1 minute.
Add the tomatoes, tomato purée and paprika. Stir for 2–3 minutes until thick.
Blend the tomato mixture in a food processor until smooth. Mix with the haricot beans, add pepper to taste and warm through over a medium heat for a few minutes.

Root Vegetable Soup

If you don't feel like spending much time preparing lunch, this is the soup for you.

2 carrots	1 tablespoon dried rosemary
2 parsnips	1 litre (1¾ pints) filtered water
1 onion	1 teaspoon ground ginger
¼ swede	

Wash all the vegetables well, cut off the ends, put everything in a saucepan whole, add water to cover the vegetables, bring to the boil and then let simmer for 15–20 minutes.

Drain, reserving the cooking water, and blend all the cooked vegetables in a food processor. Then add the reserved water until the mixture is smooth and soup-like.

Variations

For a heavier soup, add some olive oil.

You can use virtually any vegetable to make this soup. Also, experiment with different mild spices, especially garlic and ginger.

Cream of Brocolli Soup

1 head of brocolli, chopped into large florets
1 potato
120 ml (4 fl oz) soya milk

Bring all the ingredients to the boil, then simmer, covered, for 15–20 minutes.
Purée, adding more soya milk if necessary.

Variations
If you cannot eat potatoes, use oats to thicken the soup. Mix in 75 g (3 oz) of oats with the vegetables at the beginning, stir frequently while the mixture is heating to a boil, then simmer for 15 minutes and puree.
If you are allergic to brocolli, substitute a vegetable that is OK for you.

Rice Salad

This is a great dish to take to a summer afternoon party or pack for lunch. If you find you have some left over, blend in a food processor with some water and use it as a gravy.

200 g (7 oz) brown rice
500 ml (17 fl oz) filtered water
1 medium carrot, diced
½ head of brocolli, diced
1 small onion

¼ small cabbage, chopped
1 tablespoon chopped fresh
  parsley
2–3 tablespoons toasted
  sunflower seeds

Simmer the brown rice in the water, covered, for about 40 minutes. Meanwhile, boil the carrots, brocolli and onion together for 2–3 minutes. Lift them out, drain and let cool.
In the same boiling water, cook the cabbage for 1 minute. Drain and cool.
Mix all the cooked ingredients together with the rice and remaining ingredients in a bowl.

Variations
Use any vegetables you like or add cooked organic chicken for a chicken and rice salad. You can also pour Lemon, Garlic and Oil Dressing (see page 78) on top.

Quinoa Pilaf

This is a wonderful quick pilaf, very light and fluffy.

*750 ml (1¼ pints) filtered
    water
250 g (9 oz) quinoa
1 leek, finely chopped*

*1 carrot, grated
1 red onion, sliced
1 tablespoon fresh parsley,
    finely chopped*

Heat the water in a pan. Add the quinoa and leek just before the water boils. Cover and simmer for 20 minutes.
Turn off the heat and add the carrot, red onion and parsley. Let sit, covered, for 5 minutes.

Variations
Substitute any grain you like instead of quinoa.
Put in cooked chickpeas, for a nutty taste, or add toasted sesame seeds.

Workday lunches
- *Jacket potatoes*, filled with candida-friendly foods, like a tin of tuna. This is also great to order if you go out to a pub for a meal.
- *Sandwiches* Flat breads, like any floured tortilla or chapati, make great bread alternatives. Yeast-free soda bread is another option. Fill your sandwich with hummus, avocados, sprouts, lettuce, tofu, beans – the possibilities are endless!
- *Salad* Making a salad with different types of lettuce, adding sprouts and some toasted sunflower and pumpkin seeds is a great meal that travels well in a container. Bring along rice cakes and a spread (hummus or almond butter) and you have a meal.
- *Soups* Most workplaces have facilities to reheat food. This is one of the few times I would say be flexible and use a microwave if you have to. Your food may be less nutritious, but you will have food in your stomach and be able to continue working. Make

soup the night before and carry it in a container to work or see what soup the local take-away shop sells – vegetarian restaurants often have one vegan soup available on a daily basis. If they don't have a vegan selection, ask them if they could offer it once a week. Many restaurants like to do this sort of thing to please their customers. Bring some oatcakes with you and your meal is complete.

- *Pasta salad* There are lots of wheat-free pastas available. Healthfood shops carry rice pasta, corn pasta and even millet pasta. Cook pasta the night before you want to take it for lunch. Lightly steam assorted vegetables (don't overcook vegetables – it lowers their nutritional content) and mix with the pasta. Refrigerate. Put Lemon, Garlic and Oil Dressing (see page 78) on the pasta salad right before you're about to eat it, so the salad isn't soaked in oil. This can also be a quick meal for dinner.

DINNER

Have instant soups or take-aways been the norm in your house for the evening meal? By the end of the day, the last thing many people want to do is come home and cook dinner as you're exhausted. If you want to get better, though, you have to cook. This does not have to mean spending hours in the kitchen, preparing elaborate meals. Start slowly – cook dinners with your new foods that are similar to those you ate before you went on a candida diet. Then, when you're ready, try something new. There are so many basic meals you can create with candida foods that you and your family will enjoy the change.

Tofu Walnut Burgers

This is a great dish to serve to children.

200 g (7 oz) brown rice
1 litre (1¾ pints) filtered water
1 onion, finely chopped
2 garlic cloves
1 carrot, grated
1 tablespoon olive oil

250 g (9 oz) tofu
2 tablespoons Bragg soy
  sauce (optional)
2 organic eggs
50 g (2 oz) walnuts

Preheat the oven to 200 °C/400 °F (gas 6).
Simmer the rice in the water in a covered pan for 40 minutes.
Sauté the onion, garlic, and carrot in the olive oil for 3–5 minutes.
Place in a large mixing bowl.
Then, in a food processor, mix together the tofu, brown rice and soy
sauce, if using, until it forms a thick, smooth consistency. Add this to
sautéd vegetables and mix well. Beat the two eggs and mix them in.
Add the walnuts. The consistency should be similar to minced beef.
Form round burgers and place on a floured baking sheet. Bake in the
preheated oven for 45 minutes.

Variations
Substitute another nut for the walnuts.
   Use a different grain instead of brown rice.

Vegetable Curry

1 onion, sliced
1 tablespoon fresh grated root
*   ginger*
1 tablespoon sesame oil
1 carrot, chopped
3 potatoes, chopped
1 small cauliflower, chopped

1 medium courgette, chopped
1 teaspoon turmeric
1 teaspoon curry powder
*   (make sure it has no sugar*
*   added)*
250 ml (8 fl oz) filtered water

Sauté the onion and ginger in the oil for 1 minute.
Add the carrot and potatoes and cook for 2 minutes.
Add the cauliflower, courgette and stir. Then stir in the turmeric and curry powder and stir again, coating the vegetables with the spices. Pour some filtered water into the mixture until the curry is the right consistency. Break up the potatoes and cover, simmering until the vegetables are tender.

Variations
Add cooked chickpeas or meat for a hearty meal or try cubes of tofu.
Add cashew nuts.
Use garlic instead of ginger – or both!
Use different vegetables (leave the potato, though as it makes for a great thick, saucy consistency).

Lentil Bake

225 g (8 oz) red lentils, soaked
    overnight
500 ml (17 fl oz) filtered water
1 carrot, grated
1 parsnip, finely chopped

1 onion, finely chopped
5 tablespoons wholemeal
    flour
2 organic eggs
1 garlic clove

Preheat the oven to 200°C/400°F (gas 6).

Cook the lentils in the water for 15–20 minutes, until the water has been absorbed.

In a bowl, mix the cooked lentils with the remaining ingredients. Put the mixture in a floured 450-g (1-lb) loaf tin and bake in the preheated oven for 30 minutes.

Variations

If you're allergic to wholemeal flour, use any flour you can eat. Alternatively, put in 200 g (7 oz) of well-cooked brown rice instead of flour.

Use any mild spices you can tolerate.

Instead of a bake, form the mixture into burgers, coat with flour and bake for 20–25 minutes.

Tim's Shepherd's Pie

*200 g (7 oz) potatoes,
    chopped
1 large onion, chopped
100 g (4 oz) soya margarine,
    unhydrogenated
1–2 tablespoons soya milk
2 carrots, sliced thinly*

*2 garlic cloves, crushed
250 g (9 oz) minced lamb or
    vegetarian mince
100 g (4 oz) butter beans,
    cooked
250 ml (8 fl oz) yeast-free
    vegetable stock*

Preheat the oven to 200°C/400°F (gas 6).

Boil the potatoes until they are soft.

Meanwhile, gently fry the onions in all but 40 g (1½ oz) of the margarine until they are soft.

Drain the potatoes and put the remaining margarine and the soya milk in with the potatoes and mash until smooth.

Add the carrots and garlic to the onions and fry for 1–2 minutes.

Add the minced lamb or vegetarian mince, butter beans and the vegetable stock. Boil for 10 minutes for the vegetarian mince or 20 minutes for the minced lamb. Pour into a casserole dish and cover with the mashed potatoes. Bake in the preheated oven for 30 minutes or until the potatoes have browned nicely.

Variations

Use green lentils instead of vegetarian mince.

Use the bean of your choice.

Grate soya cheese on top, for extra flavour.

If you are sensitive to potatoes, substitute Millet 'Mashed Potatoes' (see page 73).

Add any fresh herbs you like. Chopped rosemary is delicious in this dish.

Lemon Gingered Chicken

6 lemons
4 organic chicken joints
1 tablespoon freshly grated root ginger

Preheat the oven to 200°C/400°F (gas 6).

In a casserole dish, squeeze the juice of 3 of the lemons over the chicken.

Thinly slice the other 3 lemons, leaving the rind on. Put the lemon slices over the chicken joints in the casserole dish.

Grate the ginger and pour the juice from the ginger (including the grated bits) over the chicken. Bake in the preheated oven for 1½ hours.

Variations

Add mild fresh herbs.

Add a little soya milk and flour to the lemon juice to make a richer sauce.

Replace the ginger with garlic or use both!

Vegetable and Millet Casserole

375 g (13 oz) millet
1 carrot, sliced
1 onion, chopped
1 tablespoon dried rosemary
900 ml (½ pints) filtered
  water

200 g (7 oz) tofu
4 tablespoons olive oil
2 garlic cloves, crushed
750 g (1½ lbs) spinach

Preheat the oven to 220°C/400°F (gas 6).
Combine the millet, carrot, onion and rosemary in a casserole dish with the filtered water. Cover the casserole dish and bake in the preheated oven for 45 minutes.
Meanwhile, cut the tofu into large, thin slices and lightly fry them in the olive oil. Remove them from the oil, drain on paper towel to remove any excess oil and let cool.
In the same pan, leaving only a little olive oil in the pan, lightly fry the garlic with the spinach for a few minutes, until cooked. Add a little water to the pan during frying to prevent the spinach from burning. Place the spinach on the side until the casserole has cooked. The casserole is done when all the water has been absorbed. When done, take the casserole out of the oven, remove the cover and place a layer of tofu on top and then the spinach. Return to the oven and bake for 5–7 minutes, uncovered. Then enjoy with Tahini Sauce (see page 77).

Variations
Steam sweet potatoes, mash them and add it as the layer before the tofu, once the casserole has baked.
Add any herbs or ginger, which is especially good.

VEGETABLE SIDE DISHES

Did you grow up eating vegetables that were boiled to oblivion? Do you still boil your vegetables to oblivion because it's just 'easier'? Well, there are alternatives to boiled vegetables! The recipes that follow are some creative ways to cook vegetables that are not very time-consuming and can pull you out of a boiled vegetable rut. If none of them suit you, try steaming vegetables instead of boiling, or boiling for only a very short time, a much better way to quickly cook your vegetables and keep the nutrients in.

Millet 'Mashed Potatoes'

If you are sensitive to potatoes, this is the dish for you. It tastes so much like mashed potatoes, you won't believe there aren't potatoes in the recipe!

> *1 litre (1¾ pints) filtered water*
> *250 g (9 oz) millet*
> *1 small cauliflower*

Bring the water to the boil, add the millet and cauliflower, cover and simmer for 25 minutes. Blend in a food processor, adding water if necessary, to achieve the consistency of mashed potatoes.

Variations
You could use potatoes instead of cauliflower if you can eat them (use 4 potatoes, peeled and diced).
Add any herbs.
Add a little soya milk and soya margarine.
Add 120 ml (4 fl oz) soya milk mixed with 2 tablespoons tahini, for a richer flavour.

Baked chips

3–4 medium potatoes, cut into chip shapes
1 tablespoon oil

Preheat the oven to 200°C/400°F (gas 6).
In a bowl, coat the chips with the oil. Put them on a baking sheet in a single layer. Bake in the preheated oven for 35–40 minutes. Turn the chips several times while baking so they cook and brown evenly.

Variations
Use sweet potatoes instead of white potatoes. Not only do sweet potatoes have a wonderful natural flavour, but very few people have allergic reactions to sweet potatoes. Check them after 25 minutes, though, because they usually take less time to cook than white potatoes.

Brussel Sprouts with Chestnuts

This is a wonderful, rich dish.

>*350 g (12 oz) chestnuts in their shells*
>*filtered water as required*
>*2 tablespoons unhydrogentated soya margarine*
>*500 g (1 lb 2 oz) Brussels sprouts*

Boil the chestnuts, unpeeled, in water to cover for 10 minutes, until the shells feel soft and loose. Take the shells off the chestnuts.
Warm the soya margarine in a pan, add the Brussels sprouts and cook for 10 minutes.
Add the chestnuts, stir and cook for another 5 minutes, or until the Brussels sprouts are cooked.

Variations
If you are able to include some fruit in your diet, try green grapes instead of or in addition to the chestnuts.
Use oil instead of soya margarine.

Nori Rolls

This dish impresses everyone. It looks like sushi and tastes great. You can take it to a party, sliced, or take it whole for lunch. Once you get the hang of it, it's very easy to make.

filtered water as required
½ carrot, cut in thin strips
3 brocolli florets, cut into strips
1 sheet of nori (dried seaweed, available from healthfood shops)

200 g (7 oz) cooked, cooled brown rice
100 g (4 oz) toasted sesame seeds
1 spring onion, halved lengthways

Boil the water and cook the vegetables in it for 1–2 minutes. Then, drain the vegetables and let them cool.

Place the nori on a flat surface. Spoon the rice onto the nori. Wet your fingers and press the rice evenly, very flat, over three quarters of the nori, leaving the quarter along the top edge empty. About 2.5 cm (1 in) up from the bottom edge of the nori, sprinkle 1 teaspoon of the sesame seeds along in a line. Then lay out each vegetable lengthwise, one at a time, in strips on top of the sesame seeds. Lift the nori from the bottom and roll it up tightly and evenly, pressing the edge inwards. Moisten the uncovered edge of the nori with water so it will stick to the roll to seal it. Allow to rest a few minutes. Cut into 2.5-cm (1-in) slices, wiping the knife clean after each slice.

Variations
Use any vegetables, but choose ones of different colours if you can so it looks nice when you slice it.
Dip the slices in Bragg soy sauce to add extra flavour when eating.

SAUCES, DIPS, SPREADS AND STUFFING

Here are a few suggestions, but often the best sauces and spreads just happen. If you feel like experimenting, choose ingredients (combine liquids and more solid foods) that you enjoy, and then taste as you go!

Tahini Sauce

120 ml (4 fl oz) tahini
1 teaspoon sesame oil
filtered water as required

Stir the tahini in a pan over a medium heat until it is lightly roasted. Add the oil. Stir in enough water in to achieve a sauce-like consistency. Simmer for 5 minutes. Do not let it boil as the tahini will curdle.

Variations
Add crushed garlic.
Sauté an onion until soft and add it to the sauce.

Lemon, Garlic and Oil Dressing

120 ml (4 fl oz) olive oil
juice of $^1/_2$ a lemon
1 garlic clove

In a small, screw-top jar, mix the olive oil and lemon juice. Add the garlic, leaving the clove whole. Shake and let sit for 5 minutes. If you put it in the refrigerator it will keep for a couple of days.

Variations
Use a different oil.
Add fresh herbs.
Don't use garlic or add chopped up parsley to counteract the garlic taste in your mouth (if you add parsley, use the dressing right away as it does not keep well).

Avocado and Tofu Spread

1 ripe avocado, stoned and flesh scooped from skin
200 g (7 oz) tofu
juice of 1 lemon
filtered water as required

Mash the avocado flesh with the tofu in a bowl. Add the lemon juice and mix well. Blend in food processor until smooth, adding water if necessary.

Variations
Add more water to make a sauce, less if you want a spread.
Throw in a clove of garlic to give it extra zing.

Hummus

Hummus is excellent for any occasion – as a dip for parties or spread in a sandwich. Plus, it's full of protein.

400 g (14 oz) dried chickpeas   *juice of 2 lemons*
2 litres (3¹/₂ pints) filtered   *50 ml (2 fl oz) olive oil*
  water   *120 ml (4 fl oz) tahini*
3 garlic cloves   *filtered water as required*

Soak the chickpeas in water overnight. The next day, simmer the chickpeas in the filtered water for 1–2 hours, until they are soft. Let cool.

Put all the ingredients, except the tahini and water, into a food processor and purée. Then add the tahini. Add water, if necessary, to create a smooth consistency.

Variations
Don't be afraid to add more of the main ingredients to make the hummus taste how you like it.

Add fresh herbs.

Use an avocado to make Avocado Hummus.

You can replace the chickpeas with tofu and create a Tofu Hummus.

White Sauce

2 tablespoons soya margarine
2–3 tablespoons flour
750 ml (1¼ pints) soya milk

In a pan, melt the soya margarine. Remove the pan from the heat, add the flour and mix to a smooth paste. Add the soya milk slowly, stirring frequently. Keep stirring while you bring the mixture to the boil, then simmer for 2–3 minutes. Add more soya milk, if necessary, to achieve a smooth consistency.

Variations
Add fresh herbs.
Substitute a different milk, like oat milk, for the soya milk.

Creamy Leek Sauce

2–3 leeks, chopped into 1-cm ($\frac{1}{2}$-in) thick slices
3 teaspoons olive oil
filtered water as required

Steam the leeks for 10–12 minutes, until soft. Transfer the slices to a food processor, add the olive oil, 2 tablespoons of water and purée for 1 minute. Add more water, if necessary, until you have a smooth sauce consistency.

Variations
Add herbs.
Add garlic.
Mix in soya milk instead of water.

Baked Garlic

For garlic lovers only! After you bake it, it spreads like butter, so use it on yeast-free breads or vegetables.

> *4 garlic cloves*
> *2–3 teaspoons olive oil*
> *120 ml (4 fl oz) filtered water*

Preheat the oven to 200°C/400°F (gas 6).
Remove the outer papery skin of the garlic and trim off the ends. Place the whole cloves of garlic in a baking dish. Pour the olive oil over them. Cover and bake in the preheated oven for 20 minutes. Add the water and baste the garlic, then continue to bake, covered, for 1 hour until the garlic is very soft when pierced with a fork.

Variations
Add any herbs and freshly ground black pepper.

Brown Rice Stuffing

400 g (14 oz) brown rice
1.5 litres ($\frac{1}{2}$ pints) filtered
  water
1 large onion
1 garlic clove
1 tablespoon oil

4 tablespoons filtered water
1 yeast-free vegetable stock
  cube
200 g (7 oz) chestnuts
parsley, chopped

Simmer the brown rice in the water, covered, for 40 minutes.
Preheat the oven to 200°C/400°F (gas 6).
Sauté the onion and garlic in the oil until soft.
Pour in the water, dissolve the vegetable stock cube in it and simmer
for 2 minutes.
Take the chestnuts out of their shells (boil them until soft and then
the shells will come off easily), chop and mix them in a bowl with all
the other ingredients. Purée in a food processor – the consistency
should be like stuffing. Bake in an oiled baking dish, covered, in the
preheated oven for 30 minutes or use to stuff a chicken and cook for
the time and the temperature that is right for its size.

Variations
You can change any of the ingredients to make a savoury stuffing.
Replace the brown rice with a different grain – maybe couscous or
millet.
Add any herbs you like.
Choose a different nut – like walnuts or pine nuts – if you don't like
chestnuts.
Add more oil for an extra moist taste.

YEAST-FREE BREADS

You can eat yeast-free breads. Right now you may think you could never give up your toast, but yeast-free bread alternatives can also be delicious. Read through the recipes below, for some fun ideas on making your own yeast-free bread.

Tortillas

These are great fresh, used to make a sandwich, or make a lot on a day you have extra time and freeze them – they'll reheat in the oven in less than five minutes.

> *175 g (6 oz) flour*
> *120 ml (4 fl oz) filtered water*
> *1 teaspoon sunflower oil*

Mix the flour, water and oil together until the dough clumps together in a ball. Break off small balls of dough and, on a floured board, knead until soft. Then, one at a time, roll out the ball of dough with a rolling pin until it is like a pancake. Flour both sides of the tortilla and bake in a hot pan, about 3 minutes on each side (you do not need oil in the pan).

Variations
Experiment with different flours.

Coconut Bread

This is delicious fresh and also freezes well.

150 g (5 oz) desiccated coconut
300 g (11 oz) wholemeal flour
350 ml (12 fl oz) warm filtered water
1 teaspoon sunflower oil

Mix the coconut and flour in a bowl and make a well in the centre. Add the warm water and mix gently.

Heat the oil in a pan, distributing the oil evenly. Drop 4 or 5 heaped tablespoons of the batter into the hot pan, leaving adequate space between each spoonful. Flatten each one with a spatula until it is no more than 7.5 cm (3 in) in diameter and 5 mm ($\frac{1}{4}$ in) thick, and cook for 3–4 minutes, until brown on the bottom. Turn them over and cook 3–4 minutes longer. Let cool. Repeat with the remaining batter.

Variations
Use soya margarine instead of oil.
Try soya milk instead of water.

DESSERTS

While sugar and its cousins may remain a 'no-no' for a while, there are still some desserts you can eat.

Carrot Pudding

400 g (14 oz) carrots, grated
750 ml (1¼ pints) soya milk
1 teaspoon grated fresh root ginger
1 teaspoon sunflower oil

In a pan, mix the carrots, soya milk and ginger, cover and simmer over a very low heat for 1–1½ hours, stirring occasionally, until the liquid evaporates. Then, in a clean pan, heat the oil and spoon in the carrot mixture, sautéing it. The mixture is wet, but will dry out as you sauté. Stir continually to prevent it sticking. Cook for 5–10 minutes. Spoon into a serving dish.

Variations
If your candida isn't too bad, add raisins or walnuts.

Baked apples

This is a treat you can eat when you feel better.

> *4–6 apples*
> *150 g (5 oz) raisins*
> *100 g (4 oz) walnuts*
> *2 tablespoons tahini*
> *juice of 1 lemon*

Preheat the oven to 180°C/350°F (gas 4).

Core the apples and pierce with a fork to prevent the skins bursting during cooking. Place the apples in a baking dish. Mix the raisins, walnuts, tahini and lemon in a bowl. Spoon the filling into the centre of the apples. Cover with foil and bake for 30 minutes. They're ready when you can pierce them easily with a fork.

Variations
Add vanilla, if you can tolerate it.
Use some ginger.
Substitute any dried fruit or nuts for the raisins and walnuts.
Eliminate all dried fruit and nuts and fill the apples only with tahini.

Sesame Oatcakes

300 g (11 oz) oat flour
100 g (4 oz) toasted sesame seeds
85 ml (3 fl oz) olive oil
85 ml (3 fl oz) filtered water
1 teaspoon sesame oil

Preheat the oven to 170°C/325°F (gas 3).
Mix the flour and seeds together. Stir in both the oils and water. Mix thoroughly. Roll out on a baking sheet with oiled wax paper laid over the dough. Cut into squares with a knife. Bake for 10–12 minutes, until lightly brown.

Variations
Use any flour instead of oat flour.
Eliminate the sesame seeds and you have plain oatcakes!

SNACKS

Here are a few ideas for delicious snacks.

- *Toasted sunflower and pumpkin seeds* In a dry pan, cook some seeds over a medium-high heat, stirring until they smell toasted. Let cool.
- *Popcorn* If you are not allergic to corn, this is a great snack. Do not use microwave popcorn (see page 44). You can pop your own by putting 1 tablespoon of oil and 200 g (7 oz) of corn kernels in a heavy bottomed pan, covering the pan and cooking over a high heat, shaking it periodically and making sure some air is allowed to escape. The popcorn is ready in 5 minutes.
- *Brown rice cakes* Or any other grain rice cake. These are available in healthfood shops.
- *Raw vegetable sticks* These are great to bring to work or eat at home, dipping them into hummus.
- *Oatcakes* Buy only those that have no added malt.
- *Crisps and corn chips* You can eat small amounts of any brands without artificial flavourings.
- *Ryvitas.*

QUICK MEALS

If you want a nutritious meal in a hurry try:

- Root Vegetable Soup and Tortillas (see pages 61 and 85)
- salad with Tahini Sauce (see page 77)
- couscous cooked with assorted vegetables (ask in your health-food shop for gluten-free couscous)
- pan-fried fish with steamed vegetables
- pasta, steamed vegetables and Lemon, Garlic and Oil Dressing (see page 78)
- tinned tuna with pasta or brown rice and vegetables.

Keep your kitchen stocked with these nutritious foods for when you have little time or just don't feel like cooking. On days when you have more time, like Sunday, cook beans, freeze them and use them later in the week when you have little time. Freezing food for no more than two weeks, is OK. Do not reheat the food in a microwave, though!

COOKING FOR SPECIAL TIMES

You can incorporate the candida foods into your daily life and have fun, too. Once you gain some confidence with your cooking, try preparing candida foods for different occasions. Even if you contribute one dish, most people will be very interested in discovering new ways of eating.

Christmas

You *can* get through Christmas day on your new diet! Try the following menu, using the recipes mentioned in this chapter.

• Lemon Gingered Chicken or Lentil Bake (see pages 69 and 71)
• Brussels Sprouts with Chestnuts (see page 75)
• roast potatoes, parsnips and carrots
• Brown Rice Stuffing (see page 84)
• Tahini Sauce (see page 77)
• Baked Apples (see page 88)

Candida dinner parties

As mentioned in Chapter 4, having a candida dinner party can be a great way to introduce hesitant family and friends to your new foods. Here's a sample menu using recipes from this chapter.

Pre-dinner snacks:	Toasted Sunflower and Pumpkin Seeds (see page 90)
	Nori Rolls (see page 76)
Main meal:	Lemon Gingered Chicken (see page 71)
	Creamy Leek Sauce (see page 82)
	Millet 'Mashed Potatoes' (see page 73)
	steamed greens and carrots
Dessert:	Carrot Pudding (see page 87)

Theme meals

A theme meal combines your candida foods with a special focus to lighten the atmosphere. Here are a few menu suggestions for the theme meals mentioned in Chapter 4.

Mexican night

- Baked beans (see page 60)
- Tortillas (see page 85)
- brown rice
- shredded lettuce and grated carrots
- sprouts
- soya cheese

Yankee night

- Tofu Walnut Burgers (use yeast-free sodabread as a bun!) (sec page 66)
- Baked Chips (see page 74)
- assorted steamed vegetables

Picnic night

- Vegetable Soup (see page 61)
- Hummus (see page 80)
- Brown Rice Salad (see page 63)
- raw vegetable sticks
- rice cakes

6

Ways to heal beyond food?

'Most people with yeast-related problems resemble the proverbial overburdened camel. To regain your health, you'll need to unload many bundles of straw.'
William Crook, *The Yeast Connection and Women*

One day while writing this book, I was feeling low and my stomach was upset, so I called my mother. 'Nothing I am eating feels right', I told her. She suggested maybe I take the advice of Norman Cousins who, when sick with terminal cancer in hospital, refused medical treatment and said instead he wanted vitamin C and a television to watch comedy shows continually so he would laugh. After several months, to the doctors' surprise, but not to his, the cancer had gone into remission. It was the power of laughter, he said.

That night, I put away my very intense book, stopped watching programs on Bosnia or Rwanda, turned on Clive Anderson and let myself laugh and laugh and laugh. By the end of the show I felt great, my stomach pains had disappeared and I had my first peaceful night of sleep in days. The power of laughter had worked in me.

You must go beyond food. Eating foods that will starve the candida is crucial to feeling better, but so is laughter and crying and complementing your new diet with other natural remedies. Having candida can be an opportunity, not a liability. *You* can hold the reigns to your health, not your doctor or fancy medical tests. When you learn more about your body, about better nutrition and strategies that help you stay healthy, your potential to feel good becomes limitless.

Recovery is a process, not a quick fix. Think about a drive through the countryside. When you are very sick, you will not notice the trees. When you feel a little better, you notice the trees, but not the colours of the leaves. When you are closer to good health, you notice the leaves on the trees are green. At optimum health, you notice all the variations of green in the different leaves on the trees. When the colours begin to return to your life, you will know you have recovered or are on the right road to recovery.

Right now, when your candida might be at its worst, recovery may seem like a distant dream. Maybe you cannot even imagine one day feeling 'clear' and wanting to wake up in the morning. Every candida sufferer knows these feelings. The ones who change their diet, improve their nutrition and actively seek ways that will aid them in their recovery, however, do feel better.

This is your journey. The right approach to good health depends on your needs, not others. Each point below outlines different approaches to compliment a candida diet that have worked for many candida sufferers. Some have got better using just one approach, some used several approaches, but the most important thing to remember is that, in order to get rid of the candida and stay healthy, you have to cure your *whole* self – body, mind and spirit.

Five positive steps to recovery

Good health is when you are not tired all the time, you have a good appetite, you sleep well, your memory is good, you're in good humour, you don't blame others for your problems, you're honest and you have a general love of life. These qualities encompass different levels of yourself – physical, psychological, social and spiritual – so healing may require you to get involved in your recovery on many levels.

You may be asking, 'Where do I begin?' When you have candida, just physically taking a step out of the door can sometimes be difficult and bring anxiety. The list that follows suggests positive steps – many of them at no financial cost to you – that you can take to get involved in your recovery.

1 Get help

Finding a caring natural health practitioner, who has experience working with candida sufferers and is willing to explain things to you, can begin the process of you feeling in control of your health. It is rare to see a doctor nowadays who has more than 15 minutes to spend with us. This is not so with most good natural health practitioners, like nutritional consultants, kinesiologists and clinical ecologists. Many of these practitioners allow for a full hour of discussion and treatment, encouraging you to ask questions and discuss issues you think are the key to your health problems. This brainstorming time can give you ideas on how to explore healing yourself on your own. It is not unreasonable to ask a lot of questions about your health – you are not a troublemaker. If the practitioner you choose makes you *feel* like a troublemaker, change practitioners. A good caring health practitioner encourages you to ask questions and is interested in you getting better, not in getting you out of their office.

You do need to seek expert help because it is generally agreed by candida experts and candida sufferers that curing yourself of candida on your own will not usually work. Of course you can find out the daily antifungal and probiotic treatments for candida, buy them and take the dose on the bottle, but you will probably be wasting your money. Many candida sufferers have tried curing themselves this way, getting advice from books or friends and spending a lot of money on every and any supplement available. Before you go and do this, stop and ask yourself, 'Do I know what I'm doing?' If I get a severe die-off reaction, what dose should I then take? When is it the right time to stop the supplements? What vitamin supplements might my body need to get better faster? Do I know what foods I am allergic to? A skilled practitioner can help you find the answers to these questions. Use them (see the Useful addresses section at the back of this book for places to look for a practitioner).

2 *Learn to listen to your body*

Your body sends out 'I'm OK'/ 'I'm not OK' signals on a daily basis. Paying attention to these signals and meeting the needs of your body is an important way to maintain balance. The signs are often not very complicated. Are you hungry? Well, then make sure you eat. Do you have to go to the lavatory? Then, go. Are you tired? Rest. Your body knows what it needs – all you have to do is listen.

When a physical sensation arises in your body – like abdominal pain, a panic attack, a headache, back pain – stop what you are doing and listen to it. Try the 'breathe, relax, watch, allow' exercise:

- Breathe: take a few deep breaths
- relax: let your body release tension (lifting your shoulders and sighing as you let them drop will often relax the body)
- watch: observe the sensation in your body that is bothering you – how does it feel now, what does it need to feel better?
- allow: let the sensation just 'be', do not fight with it – if it wants to stay, let it, if it wants to pass, allow it to pass out of your body.

Doing this with your eyes closed makes the exercise even more powerful. This is a quick exercise, so use it often, whenever sensations hit, to stay in touch with your body on a daily basis. As a reminder to do the exercise, write the words 'breathe, relax, watch, allow' on Post-Its and stick them anywhere in your home or office where you'll see them. Even if you decide to just do the first step – to breathe – your body will thank you.

Creative visualization is another way to pay attention to your body. It is probably the best, and cheapest, way to relax and listen to your body. It is very similar to meditating – a simple technique that many people think takes some special skill but only takes the commitment to actually sit down and do it. Anybody can practise creative visualization.

In her book *The Self-healing Cookbook*, Kristina Turner suggests people do an 'Inner Balance Exercise' for 15 minutes every day when you feel physically or emotionally out of balance. An adaptation of her exercise is below. Try doing it every day, and you'll soon have an ongoing dialogue with your body and be a lot closer to opening your door to good health.

First, get comfortable. Sit or lie down and close your eyes. Let each breath relax your body and mind. Sink deep – every exhalation relaxing you more. Count backwards, slowly, from five to one. Breathe out tension. Breathe in energy. Five . . . four . . . three . . . two . . . one.

Now, think of a colour that is healing and allow that colour to enter your body, starting at your toes. As the colour moves through your body, stop when you get to a place that is painful. Focus on that area. Take as much time as you need with any area in your body that is calling for attention. Let the answers come gently, from within. Trust that you and the area you are focusing on are one entity and know the cause of your pain.

Now ask, 'How can we restore the balance in that area? What small step am I ready for?' Again, take your time. Trust your inner wisdom to guide you towards a decision that's energizing, maybe even surprising. Allow your healing colour to spread throughout every area of your body, up to your head. Then, count again from one to five. Breathe. One . . . two . . . three . . . four . . . five. Open your eyes and give yourself a hug. You deserve this kind of gentle attention every day.

---

3 Release your emotions

Do you frequently get angry with your spouse, deciding not to mention anything because 'It's not worth the aggravation'? Or are you having a silent feud with a parent, burying your feelings and being 'civil' so no one gets upset? You may think that always being in emotional control is the best way to handle most situations, but think again; stored up emotions can increase the build-up of toxins in your body and create ill health. Christianne Northrup, a gynaecologist who wrote the book *Women's Bodies, Women's Wisdom*, stresses that, 'Healing can occur in the present only when we allow ourselves to feel, express, and release emotions from the past (or present) that we have suppressed or tried to forget'. Healthy people drain their emotions often, she says, allowing 'a full emotional release so our body, mind, and spirit feel cleansed and free'.

Unacknowledged emotions can lodge themselves in your body in any place, at any time. This does not happen to some people – their bodies 'forget about it' and the emotion is released. Others 'forget about it' on an intellectual level, knowing the emotion is no use thinking about, but emotionally they are *unable* to 'forget about it,' so the emotion finds a place in the body to rest and, eventually, causes pain.

Traditional Chinese medicine believes strongly in the idea that organ imbalances and stored up emotions are directly related to each other. For example, imbalances in the bowel and lung areas usually indicate the presence of grief. A kidney imbalance indicates fear. If you go to a Chinese medicine doctor, they will probably not call your health problem candida, but describe your health in terms of energy stagnation in different parts of your body, highly influenced by your emotional state.

How, then, do you release your emotions, some of which you may be totally unaware of? There are lots of different ways to do this. Some may seem ridiculous at first, but please do try them. You must experiment to find which ways work best for you. Here are a few suggestions.

- *Sing* You don't have to be a professional singer to sing. There are more and more people beginning to study the healing power of sound. It loosens your throat area, a place that often gets 'tight' when you're not feeling well, and opens up the lymph glands, allowing toxins to be released. Pick any song you like and sing it. An even better exercise is to touch an area of your body that needs healing with one hand, think of what tune that body needs to feel better and sing that tune for a minute or more. Do this exercise as a morning and evening ritual and whenever you're feeling you need to release some toxins. Also, get your partner involved and have them touch the area of your body that needs healing and let them sing the tune with you.

- *Draw* Buy yourself some colourful markers, a special blank notebook and draw. Every day, even if it's just for a minute, draw how you feel in your notebook. Use colours and shapes to express how you feel. Draw yourself or your aches and pains. Draw until you feel you want to stop. Then look back periodically to see how you've been feeling. Many times we're shocked to see what all the emotions flowing through us on a daily basis look like.

- *Write* Starting a diary can be a wonderful way to check in with yourself and write through some of your emotions. Also, if you are angry at someone and are not able to tell them to their face, write them a letter telling them what you'd like to say to them. Don't be shy, write freely, no one will see it except you! This is a great way to let go of emotions. Reread the letter a day or two later to remind yourself of how you felt, then throw the letter away. Rip it up, burn it. Allow yourself to let go of that feeling.

- *Laugh* All too often we get up in the morning, work through the day and then go to sleep without laughing once. Laughter, like singing, is a great way to loosen up your lymph nodes and encourage all the toxins to drain. A funny TV programme or going to see a comedy routine at a nightclub can transport you away from your troubles. Look up the TV programmes that will make you laugh and set aside time to watch them. Decide to be around people who make you laugh. Laughter is contagious.

4 Make lifestyle changes

Do you hate your job? Your home? Commuting to work? Only you have the power to change the bad things in your life. Living in an unhappy situation encourages dis-ease to settle into your body.

Actively participating in your life can make a huge difference to the way you feel. Certainly by changing your diet you are actively participating in your life, but there is more to life than food. What do you want to be doing five years from now? How do you want to be feeling? Envisioning your future is the first tough step to change. Once you have a vision, then you can decide which areas of your life you intend to change. Here are a few suggestions for how to make positive changes in your life:

- Make a list of all your desires. Carry this list with you wherever you go and look at it often, allowing your list to be flexible and realizing that desires are subject to your current circumstances. When you focus on and think about your desires, good things often happen to you.
- Turn your thoughts away from negative feelings; instead, concentrate on what is working in your life.
- Appreciate what is good in your life.
- Recognize that every problem is an opportunity in disguise.

Usually, candida sufferers feel their daily life is out of balance. To modify this, you do not have to make drastic changes overnight. Be aware of what you want and go at the pace you choose towards your ideal vision. Just taking the first few steps towards change can make you feel more balanced inside. If you deny that there is anything you want to change in your life, you may be denying one of the keys to better health.

5 Gather information

There is so much information available on health, healing and candida, that your journey to good health would not be complete without reading some of the useful information out there. Learning that you're not alone in your quest for good health and that others have had similar experiences to you can give you the boost you need to remember that you *will* get better and help *is* available.

Go to a library, a bookshop, visit a friend who has an interest in health, jump on the Internet, read health-related magazines . . . There is so much you can do to get yourself better – the quicker you access these things, the better. (Look through all the information at the back of this book to get you started).

Remember, you're only human

This thought is important. Respect your limits by keeping the process of healing in perspective. There is a lot you can do to get better. Some of the things mentioned in this chapter – and in this book – could be very painful for you, so if you need to stop or need help from a friend or health practitioner, do it. You are only human.

APPENDICES
Quick list of alternative foods

Keep this list on the refrigerator, to remind yourself that there are foods you can buy that are similar to the foods you used to eat. You may not be familiar with some of the foods, but they are all available in good healthfood shops. When you shop, always read the ingredients of the foods you buy carefully to make sure you can eat them. Feel free to add any new foods to the list that you discover are great substitutes for the old foods.

Cold breakfast cereals
- Puffed brown rice
- Brown rice or millet flakes
- Kashi puffed multigrain cereal
- Shredded Wheat
- Unsweetened cornflakes

Bread
- Tortillas, chapattis (not those made with white flour)
- Yeast-free wholemeal soda bread
- Rice cakes
- Oatcakes (only the unsweetened ones)
- Yeast-free pumpernickel bread

Milk
- Unsweetened soya milk
- Oat milk
- Coconut milk
- Brown rice milk

Butter
- Dairy-free, unhydrogenated margarines
- Almond, cashew and hazelnut butters (not peanut, they can carry mould)

Sugar

- Fruits
- Use apple juice to sweeten anything
- Brown rice syrup
- Sugar-free jams

Note: For at least the first few months, everyone with candida should avoid *all* sugars. After this time, some people can slowly reintroduce sugar. When you are ready to reintroduce some sugar, it is best to try unrefined sugars.

Refined carbohydrates

These are white flour, white rice and so on.

- Whole grains, like brown rice, millet, barley, bulgar wheat, quinoa, spelt, kamut, amaranth, corn
- Potatoes
- Wholegrain pastas

Wheat and gluten

- Brown rice, millet, quinoa, spelt, kamut, amaranth, corn
- Pastas using the grains above
- Gluten-free products that do not contain ingredients you cannot eat (like sugar)

Non-organic meats, poultry and fish

- Free-range and organic meat and poultry
- Free-range and organic eggs
- Tinned tuna
- Beans and pulses
- Soya mince

Food elimination and symptom chart

The chart below gives you an idea of physical symptoms that may occur when you eliminate different foods from your diet. You will not necessarily experience every symptom on the list, but, if you do, know that most symptoms are a sign of healing and will go away when the body becomes strong again. If your symptoms persist for an unusually long period of time, or just don't feel *right*, see your health practitioner.

If you eliminate . . .	*you may feel* . . .	*for* . . .
sugar	tiredness, drowsiness, depression, feelings of alienation, lack of coordination	1–5 days
coffee	headaches, shakiness, nervousness	1–10 days
alcohol	tension, inability to relax	2–5 days or more, depending on the extent of the drinking
milk and milk products	excess mucus, possibly manifesting as sinus problems, acne, temporary cysts	starting up to 3 months after the food was stopped and then for a year or two
meats, fats, protein	foul body odour, coated tongue, feelings of being toxic, skin eruptions	varies: 1–4 weeks with a fast, 6–10 months for the deeper accumulations

Source: Annemarie Colbin, *Food and Healing*

Common symptoms that indicate you may have allergies

Reviewing your medical history from infancy to adulthood is an excellent way to get a complete picture of your health and identify allergies. Read through the list below and tick which symptoms apply to you. These symptoms are often present when you have allergies to food or something in the environment. Even if you tick just a few symptoms below and you feel bad, you should contact a qualified health practitioner for diagnosis and advice.

Symptoms in infancy and childhood

Colic as an infant
Difficulty gaining weight
Skin rashes
Frequent illnesses
Difficulty sleeping
Traditionally recognized
   allergic reactions
   (asthma, hives, etc.)
Earaches or fluid in the ears
Swollen glands
Pale face
Behavioural problems
Bedwetting (after age of 3)
Short attention span

Runny or stuffy nose
Coughing or wheezing
Muscle aches
'Growing pains'
Constipation
Diarrhoea
Dark circles under the eyes
Puffiness under the eyes
Glassy eyes after eating
Sore throat
Stomach aches
Headaches
Learning disabilities
Hyperactivity

Symptoms in adulthood

Physical symptoms

Digestive problems – gas,
    bloating, belching
Abdominal distension
Sore throat
Phlegm in throat
Coughing or wheezing
Sneezing
Rapid heartbeat after eating
Heart palpitations after eating
Muscle aches
Joint pain
Dark circles, bags or puffiness
    under the eyes
Red earlobes after eating

Watery eyes
'Sand' in the eyes
Stomach aches
Constipation and diarrhoea
Rectal itching
Stuffy or runny nose
Sinus problems
Headaches
Loss of physical coordination
Swollen joints
Difficulty urinating, water retention

Emotional symptoms

Fatigue
Drowsiness
Insomnia
Irritability
Mood swings
Depression
Crying
Anxiety

Paranoia
Schizophrenic behaviour
Tendency to get angry easily
Nervousness
Loss of memory
Difficulty concentrating

COMMON SYMPTOMS THAT INDICATE YOU MAY HAVE ALLERGIES

Symptoms related to eating

Compulsive eating
Binging
Craving specific foods, such as
  bread, ice-cream
Feeling strong aversion to certain
  foods

Certain foods improve mood
Feeling better or worse after eating
Addiction to alcohol or drugs

Family history

One or both parents having
  traditional allergies

Family members who experience any
  of the symptoms above

Source: Gary Null, *Good Food, Good Mood*

Useful addresses

Food For Life
Penthouse 5
Block 3
Portman Mansions
Chiltern Street
London W1M 1PW
Tel: 0171–487 3881

Meals suitable for candida sufferers available by mail order and
through selected outlets, so if you are too busy to cook you will
always have the right food to eat.

Revital Health Shop
35 High Road
Willesden
London NW10 2TE
Tel: 0181–459 3382
For mail order, call free on 0800 252875

A healthfood shop that provides a mail-order service. It carries a
large selection of foods suitable for a candida diet.

Natural Healthcare Limited
North Health Lane
Horsham
West Sussex RH12 4PJ
Tel: 01403 253943

A natural remedy pharmacy that carries many of the products and
books necessary for the treatment of candida and related conditions. James Quinn, the pharmacist, is extremely knowledgable on
the subject of candida and available to speak to you about your

course of treatment. There are also other trained nutritional advisors you can speak to.

The Soil Association Limited
86–88 Colston Street
Bristol BS1 5BB

This is a wonderful organization to join if you want to learn more about organic food and where you can buy it in the UK. The Association produces excellent publications, including their member's magazine, *Living Earth*.

Candida Support Groups UK
Lesser Halings
Tilehouse Lane
Denham
Middlesex UB9 5DG

Find out about Candida workshops demonstrating how to cook candida recipes and introducing different therapeutic approaches to getting rid of candida. Send a SAE to the address above for more information. Also available is a listing of candida practitioners in the UK, the opportunity to find a candida support group near you, and information about their Internet page.

Action for ME and Chronic Fatigue
PO Box 1302
Wells
Somerset BA5 2WE

This is a charitable trust that provides support to people with ME and chronic fatigue and their families. Information on candida is also available.

The Wholistic Research Company
Bright Haven
Robin's Lane
Lolworth
Cambridge CB3 8HH
Tel: 01954 781074

This company can supply you, via mail order, the essential equipment you'll need for good health. Juicers, water filters, ionizers and so on. Ring for a list of items they sell.

British Acupuncture Council
Park House
206–208 Latimer Road
London W10 6RE
Tel: 0181–964 0222

Acupuncture is based on the principle that illness is the result of a blockage in the energy paths of the body. To restore the proper energy flow, restoring health, acupuncturists use fine needles inserted into specific points on the body and/or moxa herbs. For a list of acupuncturists call or write to the Council.

McTimoney Chiropractic Association
21 High Street
Eynsham
Oxfordshire OX8 1HE
Tel: 01865 880974

This is a gentle, whole body manipulation method. Call or write for more information and a practitioner near you.

British Association for Applied Chiropractic
The Old Post Office
Cherry Street
Stratton Audley

Nr Bicester
Oxfordshire OX6 9BA
Tel: 01869 277111

A manipulative therapy to treat disorders of the joints and muscles. Call or write for a practitioners' list and more information.

Colonic International Association
16 New England Lane
London NW3 4TG
Tel: 0171 483 1595

Some candida sufferers find this method a very effective way of cleaning out the toxins in their colon. Call or write for more information.

Society of Homoeopaths
2 Artizan Road
Northampton NN1 4HU
Tel: 01604 21400

Homoeopaths treat patients on the basis that 'like cures like', so they use small doses of natural remedies to restore health that in larger doses would produce similar symptoms. Call or write for more information and a list of practitioners.

Association for Systemic Kinesiology
39 Browns Road
Surbiton
Surrey KT5 8ST
Tel: 0181–399 3215

Kinesiologists use muscle testing to detect and rectify energy blockages and imbalances, which they believe are the cause of illness. They give dietary advice, too. Call or write for more information and a list of practitioners.

Society for the Promotion of Nutritional Therapy
PO Box 47
Heathfield
East Sussex TN21 8ZX
Tel: 01435 867 7007

Nutritionists use diet and supplements to restore health. Seeing a good nutritionist is often the first step most candida sufferers will take to get better. The Society has a list of nutritionists (you can also get help finding the right nutritionist from other organizations, such as All Hallows House, page 110).

Osteopathic Information Service
PO Box 2074
Reading
Berkshire RG1 4YR
Tel: 01734 512051

Osteopaths use manipulation, massage and stretching techniques to restore health. Call or write for more information and a list of practitioners.

The Shiatsu Society
5 Foxcote
Wokingham
Berkshire RG11 3PG
Tel: 01734 730 836

A shiatsu massage works on the body's pressure points to release toxins and balance your flow of energy. Call or write for more information and a list of practitioners.

Register of Chinese Herbal Medicine
PO Box 400
Wembley
Middlesex HAG 9NZ

Chinese medicine works on the principle that in order to feel good, the flow of Chi (energy) in your body must be in balance. Send an SAE and £2.50 for more information and a list of practitioners.

The British Wheel of Yoga
1 Hamilton Place
Boston Road
Sleaford
Lincolnshire NG34 7ES
Tel: 01529 306 851

Yoga is a great way to stretch your body and relax at the same time. There are many places around the UK where you can practice yoga. Write or call for more information.

Bibliography and further reading

Books:

Blythman, Joanna, *The Food We Eat*, Penguin, 1996
Chopra, Deepak, *Creating Health*, Houghton Mifflin, 1991
Colbin, Annemarie, *Food and Healing*, Ballantine, 1986
Crook, William G., *The Yeast Connection*, Professional Books, 1986
Crook, William G., *The Yeast Connection and Women*, Professional Books, 1995
Earle, Liz, *Food Allergies*, Boxtree, 1995
Haas, Elson M., *Staying Healthy with the Seasons*, Celestial Arts, 1981
Jacobs, Gill, *Candida Albicans*, Optima, 1994
McWhirter, Jane, *The Practical Guide to Candida*, All Hallows House Foundation, 1995
Northrup, Christiane, *Women's Body's Women's Wisdom*, Bantam, 1995
Null, Gary, *Good Food, Good Mood*, Dodd, Mead & Company, 1988
Stein, Diane, *The Natural Remedy Book for Women*, The Crossing Press, 1992
Trickett, Shirley, *Coping with Candida*, Sheldon Press, 1994
Turner, Kristina, *The Self-healing Cookbook*, Earthtones Press, 1987
White, Erica, *Beat Candida Cookbook*, Whites' Food Supplement Supplies, 1995 (available for £9.50 plus £1.50 postage and packing by mail order only from Whites' Food Supplement Supplies, 22 Leigh-on-Sea, Essex SS9 1RN or call 01702 72085).

Magazines:

Here's Health
Healthy Eating

Index

Recipes index